Fitness in Real Life

31 uncommonly practical lessons to make real progress in weight loss and health because real life is messy!

By: Jeremy "tall trainer" Biernat

www.talltrainer.com

Disclaimer:

This information in this book is meant to assist you not be your only resource. All exercise and health habits pose some inherent risks. Take responsibility for your own safety and health and know your limits. I'm not a doctor, nutritionist, or psychologist so please use those experts when you are not sure of something. As for any exercise and dietary programs consult your doctor before using any of these strategies.

First edition October 2016

For information about special discounts for bulk purchases or to book the author for your event, please contact Tall Trainer Fitness Systems Inc. 1(800)380-7047 or 31lessons@talltrainer.com

Cover Photo by: Amanda Lee @ www.tenfeetphoto.com

ISBN: 978-0-9980652-0-5 paperback

Dedication:

I dedicate this book to my Wife Sarah and Daughter Anna. They sacrificed the most to help me find time to write this book and I love them dearly.

I also want to dedicate this to my clients past and present as well as teachers, mentors, and my parents. I have learned all I know because of you.

Finally, I want to give God the Glory if anything in this book is helpful. He blessed me with my life, experiences, and genetics that make everything possible. It's hope in Him that keeps me moving forward.

Table of Contents

Extra Resources:

Preface

What you are about to read...

What I don't expect this book to be:
- The last information you will ever need on health, weight loss, and exercise
- Take the place of Doctors, Surgeons, Physical Therapists, Nutritionists, and Personal Trainers direct personal advice
- A one size fits all prescription. From the mental game to exercise ideas in the back, there may be things that are flat out a bad idea for you
- Every Chapter to be earth shattering amazing. Some are going to be massively helpful to you and some might be the opposite. Throw out the bad and keep the good for yourself
- Honestly I don't expect this book to be a best seller. The truth sometimes isn't glitzy, gimmicky, or shocking enough to create hysteria

I want this book to do several things:
- Be easy to read with quick and helpful chunks of information
- Be something even people who don't like to read can read (toilet length reading ;o)
- What I want people to know before training with me
- What I want people to be great at after training with me
- A way to pass on hours and hours of info in a cheap handheld package
- Be something that will remain evergreen (useful even in the future)

- Encouraging but realistic (hype free)
- Tell people what they want to know and also what they need to know
- Be a good starting point or middle point for your fitness journey
- Point you in a good direction for more information and for your next step toward a healthier and happier life

I think this book does it. While I'm sure some information will have a chance to be outdated in the future, this book is not based on current FAD diets and training principles. The majority of this information has been true for decades, centuries, and millennia. I may not tell you anything you do not know already. My goal is to help these things you already know to be put into practice more often. It may be something that you have heard before but these are some of the best ways I've ever seen to describe and demonstrate these key fitness and health concepts. Some descriptions are my own invention but I stand on the backs of giants to bring this information to you. I had to learn all this information at some point (I wasn't born knowing it). I am grateful for all my learning opportunities and I hope I condensed them in a way that will allow you to grasp them with fewer hours, weeks, and years of study than I have undergone.

I know this will also not be my "last word" on fitness and health as there are some ideas I didn't include because of length and keeping this book un-intimidating. Also, as long as I am alive I hope to be learning and growing more. I may even find better ways to explain these things in the future and have new ideas to experience. I hope you enjoy this book and if only one of these ideas is truly helpful I believe that will be enough to make it WELL worth your time.

How to read this book:

- If you are antsy for momentum in your fitness and health you can go to the back and check out the quick start guide. You can start implementing some activity and awareness before you start the first chapter.

- Commit to read one chapter per day. There are 31 chapters because the longest months have 31 days - Each chapter is a self contained thought but they do work like dots that come together to create a more complete picture.

- Once you read this book once start putting the ideas in place. After a month or so bring it out again and re-read it. New ideas will surface as you will now be in a different place in your journey.

- Once you have read this book and have found it useful invite other people close to you to read it also. This will create a culture of people around you that understand and value some of the same concepts. (It will surely help them for sure but it will also help you be more successful)

1

Chairs...Your Mortal Enemy

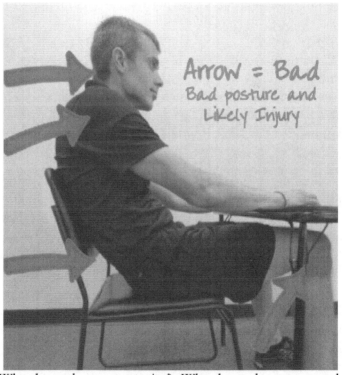

Why do we have to exercise? Why do we have to stretch?
Why do we have such terrible joints? Foam rolling doesn't
seem like God's plan.

One of our three parts to our basic philosophy is to move
the way God designed us to move. (The other two are eat
the way God designed us to eat and to strive to be better

not for perfection). Exercise for exercise sake doesn't seem like it's God's plan. I agree, but there are about a million others things that we do that don't match up with this plan also. Sitting for hours and hours is one of these things.

Research is coming out how a days worth of sitting is about as bad for you as smoking! We drive long commutes to work. Sit at work. Drive home. And after a day of sitting we don't have much energy we need a break so we sit in front of the TV.

This starts early. We start people off at 5 and 6 years old sitting for long periods of the day. Through our school years our bodies are already shaping to the chairs. The increase in non-contact ACL tears in athletes can be attributed in part to this sitting then trying to participate in sports. You wonder why it's so hard to get kids to sit still? Maybe we aren't designed to!

Bathroom/doing your business/elimination isn't even best performed sitting. A squat is more physiologically benefitial than sitting. Don't agree check out this awesome and funny product www.squattypotty.com.

Free time is now spent sitting too. With hours and hours per day of TV watching being attributed to the average American. For some if there isn't a computer (sitting), phone, (often sitting), or TV (sitting) they aren't sure what to do with themselves.

What does sitting do?

Remember when your mom told you, "don't make that face for too long or too often or it will get stuck that way!" Well she's right on a very basic principle. Our bodies will adjust to our habits. Even our bones begin to calcify and shape in response to load. (Even poor posture). While it might be tough to put in the hours to get your face to stick that way, it's fairly easy to put in the hours to get your body to get stuck in poor posture.

Poor Posture Caused by Sitting

Bad Posture	Effect	Likely Long Term Effects
Neck – Chin Sticks Out	Back of neck muscles tighten, spasm, hurt, and can cause nerve impingement.	Migraines, unbearable neck pain, herniated disc, surgery, numbness in hands.
Shoulders – Round Forward (slouch)	Shoulder range of motion decreased, increase likelihood of rotator cuff tear, increase impingement of nerves to arms and hands.	Rotator Cuff Tear, Neck pain, Numbness in hands/arms.
Lower Back – Bent Forward	Discs are loaded and ready to rupture and herniate at slightest movement.	Back injury, surgery, limited ability, pain, etc.
Hips and Calves – Locked in Place and Lose Flexibility	This puts additional pressure on the low back and the knees to perform the extra motion during movement and activity.	Knee Pain, Early wear on knee, knee replacement, Back injury, plantar fasciitis, etc.

So what I can't sit now?

Fitness in Real Life

Remember we strive to be better not perfect. Not sitting ever is also not a realistic solution. Here are some ideas to minimize the problems:

- A well-planned workout designed to undo some of the sitting type posture will help correct some of the non-perfection of daily life.
- An adjustable workstation would help so you can work from sitting and standing part of the day.
- Set limits on recreational TV especially with computer based job.
- Break up sitting time whenever possible (drink lots of water so you have to pee! :o)
- When running the kids around don't wait in the car get out and either stand by car (nice weather) or go inside.
- You are a creative intelligent person, I bet you can come up with more ideas.

On top of research about how sitting effects posture leading to injury there is also research that puts you as higher risk for a heart attack the more you sit. As the headlines are reporting "sitting is the new smoking." This stuff could kill you! One issue is the heart and lungs are not getting exercised when we sit ALL day. Another issue is the standing burns about 1 Calorie per minute more than sitting. Sitting burns about 1 Calorie per minute (give or take depending on the metabolism of the person) while standing is more like 2 Calories per minute. Sitting often equals weight gain and weight gain puts us at high risk too.

Imagine if you stood for even 3 hours out of 8 at work then when you got home you went for a walk everyday for an hour and then did some projects around the house instead of watching TV for another hour. You'd burn an extra 180 Calories at work, 120-240 Calories in your walk (depending on speed), and an extra 60-120 Calories in

1 - Chairs...Your Mortal Enemy

other activity around the house. Your total additional Calorie burn for the day could be 360 – 540 Calories extra per day. Done daily for a year is 131,400 to 197,100 Calories which is equivalent to 37 - 56 Pounds of Fat!!! Without adding a bunch of exercise. If you don't have any weight to lose that's up to 386 orders of large fries from a fast food place that you could eat extra without gaining weight.

I don't know about you but FREE calories sound awesome! Let's get away from those chairs. If you already have some of the effects listed in the table it's not too late to do something, but you need to get on it ASAP. Jack LaLanne is famous for saying. "The only way you can hurt the body is by not using it."

2

Are you a Yo-Yo Dieter?

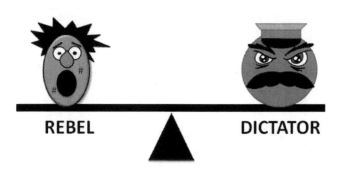

REBEL　　　　　**DICTATOR**

If you are, it is likely you are spending time on this teeter-totter with the Rebel and the Dictator. We have two opposing parts of our personality (at least two!). We have our Rational Side sometimes referred to as a Parent or Dictator. And we have our Emotional Side characterized as a Child or Rebel.

See if you can relate to this:

We go on a "diet". We lay out our rules. There will be no eating after 7 pm, no desserts, no potato chips, hardly any bread, and only good stuff for my body. We lose weight. We feel cravings but fight to keep them squashed down. If it's working this weight loss creates energy to keep to the rules. Next, we either reach our goal or get stuck at a plateau in the process. Either way the results are often the same. We are tired of the rules. We either celebrate our achievements with a break from the rules or in our plateau frustration we throw out the rules and give in to the cravings. This can last a meal or a decade. We have no limitations on food and eat whatever whenever. It's anarchy. Finally we have a sobering moment. Our clothes don't fit, we see the scale hit the high point again (or above), or our self loathing reaches a peak that we HAVE TO DO SOMETHING ABOUT THIS!!! So we bring in rules and another "diet" begins.

This ping-pong type action is very common and very frustrating. You say things like:

- Why can't I have more will power?
- I'm so weak when it comes to food.
- Why can't I ever stay at my low weight?

We think it's our non-dieting persona that is at fault for this. If only I didn't have that weakness then I could stay on my rules forever.

It's not the emotional rebel side that needs as much changing. It's the rational dictator side. How so?

Let's look at this same concept in two other scenarios. A literal dictator and rebel. Let's get political. In a dictatorship the dictator has all the power. Most often they start off beloved. They come in and fix things and make life better. Slowly the dictator's power grows and so do the abuses of that power. If the dictator limits freedom too much the people may start meeting in secret to plot against the dictator. As the abuses get greater (or go on longer) more people join the rebellion. Finally they are not meeting in secret. They now have more people behind them than the dictator and a rebellion takes place. There is fighting and if the rebellion wins they often kill the dictator. The rebellion didn't have much more of a plan beyond getting free of the dictator so the country falls into anarchy. Basic needs aren't getting met. Transportation, water, power, etc are all effected. Sometimes the country is thrown into a mini dark ages. They cry out for help. "Someone save us!" So in steps a new dictator to "save" the people and the cycle begins again.

We think to ourselves what if the dictator is super strong? Won't that stop a rebellion? What if you are a super strong and super strict "diet"er? Unfortunately, I have found most often that the stronger the dictator the bigger the rebellion. Our other scenario that is so common but can also be tragic is the parent child relationship. What if a parent is super authoritative, you know…really lays down the law? When they say jump the kids ask "how high?" Well, often these kids do test the limits at times. If you have a REALLY strong dictator…(I mean parent) they will punish and squash the rebellion out of the child. The only problem with this is eventually this child will have more freedom when they leave home. They are eagerly counting down the days like a prison sentence. They get their freedom and go do many of the things they weren't allowed to do. Sometimes to a tragic end. So, being a strong dictator is not the key.

The solution to this problem for the emotional, child, and rebel is to have a benevolent dictator/parent. If this parent type force is teaching and lifting rules as competence grows there may be nothing to rebel against. In our work to lose weight we need to have a softer approach. One of my favorite tools is the 4 F-words of diet success. (First time I heard this was in a Dr. Len Kravitz lecture he's got some gems!)

4 F-words of Diet Success:
- **Flexible** Plan – does not require perfection to work.

- Not a **Failure** if you mess up – failure is an event not a person.

- **Forgive** yourself – let the past go (even if it was 5 minutes ago).

- **Fix** – The first 3 are beautiful and lovely and necessary but without this 4th step you would still be stuck not achieving your goals. So after you forgive you then think of how you can fix your plan to make it better. This is where great leaders ask questions. How can we make this easier to do the healthy thing? How can we make the unhealthy behavior less likely? What is missing from the plan to help us feel more balanced and healthy?

This emotional rollercoaster of Yo-yo dieting is very hard to beat. Most people keep trying to beat it with the next "diet" instead of trying to figure out where this rebellion is coming from. It's like pulling weeds but they snap off at the surface level instead of getting to the root. If you have gained weight because you are coping with emotions with food you can pause it for a while and lose weight. This removes the visual evidence (extra fat) but the problem or issue is still there (roots). Eventually the roots will show themselves again.

If you don't get to the root, your problem is just going to come back later...

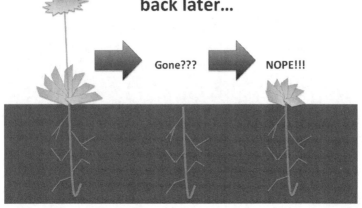

Gone???   NOPE!!!

Recommended resources to battle chronic Yo-Yo Dieting:

- Start Journaling your thoughts and ask yourself questions. It needs to be on paper because our heads are a crazy jumbled place. Writing it out organizes our thoughts. What does food do for me? What besides food could help?
- Books
  - "The Four Day Win" – Martha Beck
  - "The Gifts of Imperfection" – Brene Brown
  - "I Deserve a Donut" – Barb Raveling
  - "Boundaries" – Henry Cloud
  - "Shades of Hope" – Tennie McCarty
- Counseling – find a local counselor or see the top in the field www.interactcounseling.com

3
Habit Loop

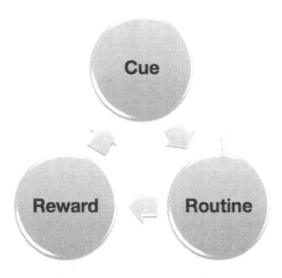

When you strip away all the complexities and get to the root of our weight loss and health struggles it's all about HABIT. We are a collection of our habits. Where we are financially is due to our habits. How much fat is on our bodies is due to habits. The little things we do everyday have a massive effect on major factors of life.

BAD and GOOD

Sometimes when you say the word habit people only think of "bad" habits. Habit can sometimes sound like a loss of control. Habits are one of the greatest time and energy savers we have. When I put on my shoes I don't have to decide which one I will put on first. I have a habit that frees my mind up to think about other things while I tie my shoes (like thinking about the next amazing workout at our studio). Habits are neither all bad nor all good. They are sometimes desirable and undesirable, and that is something each individual must decide on a habit-by-habit basis.

You Dirty Rat

Habits are like a pathway in the woods. The first time you walk that path it may not be a path. You have to clear a path as you walk it. It takes forever! After walking it daily it becomes well worn. Eventually it gets paved and becomes a road and if travelled enough becomes a super highway where you can zip to the destination with ease and in seconds instead of hours.

One study put rats in a maze and put a piece of chocolate at the end of the maze. They monitored the rat's brain activity. The first time in a maze took the rat forever. It was sniffing the air and scratching at the walls and investigating every corner. The rat's brain was going crazy processing all the information. After hundreds of times in the maze the researchers could put the rat in the maze and it would zip to the chocolate at the end of the maze with the brain hardly lighting up. That is what we call a habit. For some of us we have a habit of zipping straight to the chocolate without our brains lighting up and we don't want that habit.

The big lesson in both these examples is that habits are hard to break (like turning a super highway back to forest) and they are hard to start at the beginning (like bushwhacking through the woods). However, your new habit can become easy and near effortless in time.

Habit Loop

There are 3 parts to the habit making process. Cue, Routine, and Reward. These three factors make up the habit loop which it one of the many concepts described by Charles Duhigg in his book "The Power of Habit".

Cue	The signal to start the habit. For the rat the cue was being placed in the maze.
Routine	This is what most people refer to as "the habit". For the rat it was running the maze.
Reward	Is the incentive for completing the habit. Without an incentive the activity will never become a habit. The rat's reward was chocolate.

The more desirable the reward and the more interrupting and obvious the cue the stronger the habit. We need to consider all 3 of these parts when trying to break an undesirable habit or when trying to start a desirable habit.

Habit Breaking - To break a habit there is typically only 2 courses of action.

#1 – Disrupt the cue. If you can stop or avoid the signal to begin a habit you never even use willpower! If cookies on the counter make you eat them you'll want to move them where you don't see then as much or tell someone to stop making them (or stop making them yourself). The top expert in this area is Brian Wansink PhD. I recommend both his books mindless eating and slim by design. They are both about changing our environments to become healthier. There are hundreds of ideas in there.

#2 – Develop a new routine that supplies the same or similar reward. Once you have been cued on the habit it will fester until you get the reward. You finish a long day of work and come home walk into the kitchen and mindlessly begin to snack before dinner. What are the possible cues for this action?

Possible Cues:
1. Time of Day?
2. Where are you?
3. What Emotional State?
4. Who else around?
5. What action preceded urge?

For this example it could be time of day (after work), location (kitchen), Emotional state (tired), who else around (perhaps no one around is a cue). Whatever the cue, the trick here is to find something that TRULY does fulfill the craving. For certain habits this is hard to do. It can be helpful to think through what the cue was or what benefit you got from the old routine to help you brainstorm a new routine and reward. Let's say the main reward you were getting from the old routine was unwinding after work. A new routine could be stopping by the gym after work. Call a friend. Go for a walk outside. Stop at a park on the way home just to sit on a bench for a few minutes. Have dinner right away (have it closer to being ready). The possibilities are endless and unique as we are as people.

Habit Making - To make a habit you do the opposite of the breaking process. Two pieces most people forget when trying to start a new desirable habit are:

#1 - Creating a Cue - You won't get very far on your habit if you haven't created a consistent reliable signal to tell you to start. An example would be sleeping in your workout clothes. Then you are cued upon waking.

#2 - Designing a Reward – Sure there are intrinsic rewards to exercise and healthy eating but to create a strong habit the reward needs to happen right after the activity. Some people reward themselves for their workout by eating a treat. This can help us to keep working out but could actually cause our workout habit to cause us to GAIN weight! Make sure your reward is valuable, right after action, and doesn't conflict with your goals.

Mastering your habits is a life long process but contains the secret to more effortless success and fulfillment. I hope this sheds some light into how and why you do what you do. Now go break some habits and make some new ones!

4

Care for your body like a plant
(Moderation and Consistency)

Before I use this analogy I want you to know I'm not very good at taking care of plants. I would need a personal trainer for plant care to make sure they stayed alive.

What do plants need?	What do we need?
Good Soil and Temperature	Good Environment
Sunlight	Exercise
Water	Nutrition
Time	Time

Good Environment

Do we call a plant defective if it won't grow in frozen ground? What if it wilts in 100+ degree temperatures? If the soil is rocky? Most reasonable humans realize that those are not good environments for successfully growing a plant. There is nothing wrong with the plant it just needs a better environment to grow.

It kills me all the time when people have a terrible environment to live and work in and they blame

16

themselves for not having the willpower to break through the rocky frozen soil that is their life. It's not all you! Well, it is all you only because you chose some of that environment. When you are a child you are born into an environment that you did not choose, but as you turn 18 you begin to have the freedom to choose your own environment. If your environment stinks you can always consider transplanting yourself into a better one. If you've got that desire now, what can you do to make it better? DON'T SAY I CAN'T because that's a cop out.

What can I do to make my growing environment better?
- Change Jobs / Careers?
- Marriage Counseling?
- Move yourself and/or family?
- Join a church?
- Proactively seek out healthy friends?
- Say "no" to draining commitments?

All these are possibilities. They don't all have to be things you want to do but they are all available to you. (No "I can't") If you find some way to improve your environment and it is a big decision, get wise counsel. This is why getting fired can be the best thing to ever happen to someone. They are forced to find a better environment.

Sunlight

Plants need a balanced amount of sunlight. Too little and they are not stimulated enough to grow and too much they get burned up. When you go to the nursery and find plants for sale they often have a tag on them that describes the best growing environment. Sunlight is one of the biggest factors. Some need partial sun while others need all day. Some can get by with a very small amount but tend not to grow as fast.

We are the same when it comes to exercise. Too little and our bodies are not stimulated enough to make any positive difference. We start to waste away. Too much exercise and we begin to breakdown. When a seed is just sprouting it is more sensitive to a burning hot sun. We don't tolerate a massive amount of high level exercise very well at the start either. Give yourself enough work to begin seeing progress but not so much that you are going to hurt yourself. This is one of the benefits of working with a trainer (think expert gardener). They have seen "plants" similar to you grow many times and can balance your exercise to find that perfect zone for the level you are currently at.

Water

We all know plants need water. In fact this is probably the reason most people say they do NOT have a green thumb. They forget to water it then drown it to make up for the lack. The poor plant is either starved for water or suffocated. It dies from too little water or too much water.

We are the same when it comes to nutrition. Hitting that balance point is very tough to do. I know by experience working with thousands of people that this is a struggle. Many people will go without significant food for part of the day (or for several days) but then eat way too much later. We also know that people die from starvation as well as from obesity. It's strange that both are happening all over the world as you read this! Stranger still is they both are happening consciously by people in your town. They may not have an end goal of death but their actions will still bring about that consequence. (Some may be seeking death though and if you are feeling hopeless and using food or lack of food to disappear please get help!

4 – Care for your body like a plant

The world needs you, yes you, God has a plan for you if you'll step into it.)

We need to find the balance of food. If we have been over feeding for awhile we still need to eat but we can eat less and burn off some food from the past. If we are underfed we may need a little extra to get back to a healthy weight. If we are underfed just part of the day we need to work on spreading our food out more evenly so we spend most of the day in a healthy vibrant state.

Time

This is one of the toughest factors if you are an impatient type. I remember planting cucumbers when I was 8 or 10 years old. I would check them everyday. Nothing seemed to be happening. Yes, there was a plant there but I couldn't tell the difference day to day. I was bored and frustrated. Then we went away camping for a week and when we came back I found a cucumber! When I was staring at it daily expecting instant results I didn't notice the changes that were happening. When I gave it more time I noticed a massive change!

Our weight loss journey will be much like this. Day to day it's boring and frustrating much of the time. Without measurements that you are keeping track of it can seem like nothing is happening. You might be a pound down here or there but it just isn't fast enough! When the weeks become months and you've been consistent on the watering and sunlight you will be able to look back at the start and see a huge change! This just happened for someone yesterday. They found a picture of before they started their program with us and were shocked! They showed it to me and I was shocked! Daily the change isn't massive and some months you get stuck but if you stick to it like this person did 10 months later we are looking at

Fitness in Real Life

50+ pounds lost and nearly a completely different looking person! Give yourself patience and time as you journey to better health, fitness, and weight loss. It will come if you stay consistent on the basics, a good environment, balanced sunlight, and water. :o)

5
Working Out 101

I want to make sure you have a basic knowledge in these areas so you can get the most out of the workouts in the back of this book and ANY workout you ever do. The specifics of workout routines are to numerous to mention. These are some good over arching principles that you can apply to any workout you do. These are agreed upon by the greatest number of experts, myself included. I have tried to take some of the science jargon out of this and speak "normal human" as much as possible.

If I were starting from scratch (and many of our clients are) I would suggest this:
- If you only have minutes per day then stretch
- If you only have about 1 - 2 hours per week for exercise do resistance training
- If you have a little more time add in interval cardio training
- Then if you have more time to commit to it you can add in steady cardiovascular training

Why this order?

Most people want to start with cardio because they figure cardio will help with fat loss. It does help us burn more calories but it is not as helpful for sustained success, rebuilding metabolism, or injury prevention. Stretching needs to be first because it can increase mobility, decrease likelihood for injury, and generally make you feel younger (who doesn't want that?) Resistance training can help us build back lost muscle which will increase our daily calorie burn (resting metabolism). It also can make us more stable and strong for other activities (like cardio). Perhaps best of all it can get us leaner looking even without weight loss. I find it can have the biggest effect on someone's body and quality of life when compared to cardio. Interval training is a shorter version of cardio that can deliver a metabolism boost and cardiovascular system improvements with only a fraction of the time. Once you are limber, have strong muscles, and a boosted metabolism you may not have time for much cardio on top of that but you will already have most of the benefits that people are seeking. If you do have time then cardio can help to speed up your results with whatever time you can put in.

Resistance Training 101

I call this resistance training not weight training because you don't need to use any external weights to get a workout for your muscles. Most often people do but there are many options besides "weights." Remember I think this comes before cardio in importance. In our boot camp program we introduce resistance training by giving people an order of priorities:

#1 - Posture
#2 - Range of Motion
#3 - Extra resistance, complexity, or speed

The way priorities are supposed to work is that you NEVER compromise a #1 priority for #2. So you don't do a big range of motion if it makes you compromise your posture. Also you don't make it tougher, faster, or heavier unless posture and range of motion are amazing. These priorities help prevent injuries while you are working at that very hard level. It keeps the pressure away from the joints and allows a lighter weight to work the muscles to their maximum level.

Posture:

Ideal Posture Check Points:

- Head Back (ears over shoulders not in front of shoulders)
- Chin pulled Back (not sticking out)
- Shoulders Down away from ears and rolled back so the chest is out
- Abs Pulled in Slightly and butt tightened slightly to keep hips level (not tipping forward)
- Knees slightly bent (not hyper extended)
- Weight on heels and slightly on the outside edge of feet when standing

Range of Motion:

For most exercises there is a limited range of motion we can do while maintaining good posture. If we got beyond this point we will have to compromise posture in order to move that far. Preserving posture usually means limiting range of motion until the strength and flexibility improve enough to go farther. This is a slow process if you have had poor posture for many years. We do test the limits of posture and range of motion. When we go as far as we can in good posture we will find a stopping point or a sticking point. At this point you can feel the temptation to lose posture to make it easier, don't do it! If you can maintain posture and work into that stuck point you will slowly move that stuck point farther away. Eventually you have full range of motion and can begin loading the exercise more.

Resistance/Complexity/Speed:

These certainly should not be added all at once. They may not need to be added at all. It will depend on individual training goals. Lot's of speed is unnecessary and dangerous for most people. The exception is for sports. There will be a time and place to add speed into our movements to mimic the speed of play. An example for increasing complexity could be doing a squat on an unsteady surface once you master squats on a steady surface. For the typical person the thing we add most often is resistance. Many people do this too soon. They increase weight even before they have proven themselves at the previous weight. What typically happens is that range of motion gets smaller and posture breaks down in order to do the heavier weight. This is usually the ego getting ahead of the body. An example of this is most guys (it's usually guys) doing squats in the gym. They will put big weight on the bar but only go 1/2 way down. They are creating extra tightness that will likely become a back or knee injury someday. With resistance training we need to start humbly and focus on quality movement instead of quantity of weight.

Other principles for resistance training:
- Work on multi-joint exercises first. Squats before a leg extension.
- Most of the results and benefits come from just a couple exercises. Make sure you focus on the one's that have the biggest benefit.
- Make sure you get some of the main body movements. Squat or Bend, Pushing, and Pulling. There is bracing and rotation that are helpful too but can be added later.
- Typically it is recommended that you do two pulling exercises for every pushing exercise because of how rounded forward our posture is. This is the opposite of what many people do when they do tons of push-ups and bench presses.

- No joint pain during the exercises. If you feel joint pain stop right away. Either learn how to do it without pain (posture change or range of motion change) or get a different exercise that has similar benefits without the pain.

- Move slower to increase control and safety. There are still amazing benefits and I think more from slow repetitions than fast. Standard lifting tempo is considered 3 seconds down and 1 second up. Even that is slower than most people lift. Want to try something extreme? Try 10 second repetitions…whoa…you don't need much weight for that!

- If you aren't familiar with resistance training I would get a trainer a couple times a week for at least a month to lay a good foundation for you. I "winged" it and ended up hurting myself too many times. It's worth the investment.

Cardio Training 101

FITT – Frequency, Intensity, Time, and Type are some of the key variables in cardiovascular training. Frequency is how often or how many times per week. Intensity is how hard you are working often described as a heart rate level or a level of perceived exertion. Time is the duration of each session. Type is the kind of exercise you are doing. The main types are running, biking, and swimming but there are thousands of activities that can get the heart rate up.

Interval Training – I would start with interval training. It has been shown to have the highest benefit compared to time spent. It is the most intuitive type of training because this is how kids naturally play. I remember back in my student teaching (Elementary PE) I had the unique joy of sending a herd of kindergarteners to try a lap on a track occasionally. It was one of the most wonderful things I have seen in my life! They LOVE it for starters! It's not until we are older that we hate moving. Moving is exciting for them because they've been getting better and better at it since they were born. They are their fastest in their little lives right then! They all take off running hard with a big smile on their faces. Then after about 10 seconds some start walking (still smiling). When another kid runs by they often start to run again then stop again, run again and stop again. They must do it 10x or more in that one lap on the track! They also play like this on the playground. If you look at the whole playground it looks like every kids is going NUTS non-stop. Not true however. If you pick out one kid to watch you will see them speed up and slow down. They will run somewhere then stop and look around. We could learn a lot from this habit. The majority of our cardiovascular training in our fitness boot camp program is considered Interval Training. Once people have gotten through a few workouts we introduce high intensity interval training, which takes the heart rate up higher for a moment and often has a more dramatic rest time.

Examples of interval training are:
1 minute on 1 minute rest
20 seconds on 10 seconds rest
30 seconds on 1 minute rest

There are countless possibilities with timing and rest intervals. You need to change it up to challenge yourself differently but also know what benefit you are going for. My favorite information to learn in college was the energy systems of the body because it helps you to understand what you can expect in your performance during interval training.

When going as hard as you can this is what is happening:

- 0-10 seconds – Our bodies use a quick energy system that uses stored energy in the muscles called (ATP) – You don't typically feel the "burn" yet and you can really go fast!

- 10-20 seconds – We start to have to make more energy so extra work begins happening. You can still go fast but you start to feel some "burn".

- 20-30 seconds – Somewhere in here you will start to slow down (even if you don't want to). The "burn" will get pretty intense and you'll notice you are breathing super hard.

- > 30 seconds – You will need to slow down because your body cannot keep up with that high a level of energy usage.

If you are planning a workout do not plan on going at your top intensity over 30 seconds. You just physically can't do it! Exercise Intervals over that number it is understood that you will be pacing yourself. Using a high intensity perhaps but not your highest. Rest break is a big factor that will determine if you can do that again. These rest intervals also work well in resistance training also.

Rough % recovery over time:

1 minute – 50% recovered
2 minutes – 75% recovered
3 minutes – 90% recovered
5 minutes – 95%+ recovered

This of course depends on a lot of factors but it can be helpful frame of reference as you plan what you want to do. An example of an interval routine we have used was 30 seconds all out hard and resting for about 2 minutes repeated for 4 sets. With that I expect that the performance will drop with each attempt even in the highest trained. What I see happen a lot in fitness classes is an instructor or trainer will be trying to get people to go to their hardest level with less than a minute recovery. It just won't happen and it's not because someone is un-motivated. It just isn't physiologically possible. When trying to repeat a maximal performance you will be needing closer to 5 minutes rest to have any kind of shot at it.

Safety:

I recommend not doing ANY cardiovascular exercise alone if you can avoid it. But, certainly make sure you do interval training around others. Well fed and well hydrated are important factors in having a good experience (ie. not getting too nauseous). I want others around because if you have a problem there is someone there who can help. They don't happen all the time (never had one in my training center) but heart attacks do happen. Early care is essential. That being said I recommend starting your workout program with a trained expert to make sure you progress properly.

High intensity interval training with the wrong exercises can be very dangerous for the average exerciser. You need to choose exercises that your body can handle and don't create too much impact or stretch if your body isn't ready yet. In our program we work with people who have been out of the exercise game for decades (or have never done any). We don't do much running. For someone untrained it is a bad idea to try running hard and fast until much later (if ever). We use a stationary bike (Schwinn Airdyne or Air Assault Bike). On a bike the range of motion is controlled and impact is almost non-existent. I recommend this as a starting point for most interval training.

Duration:

5 – Working Out 101

Interval training workouts can be as short as 4 minutes (your could argue shorter too) to 45 minutes for athletes. For endurance athletes like marathoners they might go longer than the 45 minutes because they are training for a LONG sporting event.

NON- INTERVAL CARDIO SPECIFIC ADVICE:

Some of what we already covered about interval training can help as you understand non-interval cardio. I sometimes classify this as get up and move exercise! It doesn't need to be killer. The most important part of this is the duration. As humans we just need to be more active. Going for a walk, hike, bike ride, kayaking, snow shoeing, or window shopping on main street. The more time you spend off your butt the better.

Intensities:
Low – Easy to have a conversation
Medium – Broken conversation
Hard – No conversation possible (don't bother me I'm trying to breathe)

This can happen at any speed you could be slowly walking and at a hard level if it is up a mountain! Most of your cardio should be done at easy or medium. High intensity intervals will be at the hard level but for only up to minute at a time usually.

Specific recommendations:
- Don't do too much too soon – most people decide walking is lame so they try running but they go too hard and too far and end up injured.
- Choose something you enjoy – make sure this is something you like to do. If not you won't want to do it often and you'll be looking for a "reward" when you finish.

29

- Lay the foundation with stretching, resistance training, and interval training first.
- For general awesome health you can do pretty well with 1 plain cardio day per week. (If it's just get up and move you can do that for hours every day!)
- It can be over done – don't try to work at your hardest level 5 days per week for over 30 minutes per day. If you are going to do that much take the intensity back to a conversational level.

Stretching 101

Flexibility is a key component to "feeling" younger. I remember in college I got so tight that it felt like I needed to warm-up for 45 minutes before I could sprint. I almost constantly felt like something was about to pull. When I learned the value of stretching I began to feel more childlike, as if I could take off and run at anytime I desired. Do you think Yoga has a big following by accident? They are basically stretching for 60 minute sessions sometimes. Done right that can feel amazing! There is a set of stretches you can learn in the back of the book but just like the resistance and cardio sections I want to give you some big tips that will help you in all your stretching and flexibility activities.

Strengthen and Stretch - The best stretching we do with our clients is the resistance training. Proper posture and range of motion in resistance training stretches while it strengthens the right parts of your body. Proper posture is the key here to get the flexibility in the correct places. This is one of the reasons the squat exercise was so powerful in helping me heal my back. It did and still does stretch my hips out so much that my back gets less pressure throughout the day.

5 – Working Out 101

Pre-workout – Active dynamic full body movements are the best way to warm-up and get ready for exercise. We do the same warm-up daily in our classes.

End of workout - Static stretching (holding stretches for a period of time) is better used at the end of a workout.

Gaining Flexibility – Stretching needs to be done daily and positions need to be held for a while. 30 seconds holds are what we do at the end of workouts but this is more of a maintenance level. If you need to GAIN flexibility time intervals can get to holding stretches for 2 minutes or more.

Stretching Pain - this one is tricky for me because it is painful to do a good stretch. In high school I was taught not to stretch to the point of pain and that made me crippled tight by college. Since then I realize it is quite uncomfortable to stretch and if you know where you are supposed to feel it you can do it pretty hard. Moderate stretch held for long durations may be the key to long lasting flexibility. Make it personal, if it feels too hard like you are pulling something back off a little and hold longer. As long and you move slowly and carefully into the stretch the danger level is lower. If you jump into a stretch fast you certainly have a good chance to tear something. I recommend learning stretching with a professional so they can talk you through it.

Self-Myofascial Release - (Foam Rolling) I have had great benefit from foam rolling when I have a particular cranky spot. I find it works best for back pain, knee pain, and foot or achilles pain.

PNF (proprioceptive neuromuscular facilitation) - This is often done with a partner and follows a stretch, contract, relax pattern. You get into a stretch your partner holds the stretch still while you flex like you are trying to push out of it. After a few seconds you relax and try it again. I have gained the most flexibility in the shortest time using this method. The only problem I see with this one is you REALLY need to trust your partner since they have you in a vulnerable spot.

Other sections of this book that cover posture and injuries will talk a little more about stretching that I don't want to repeat here. Also, check the back section for a stretching routine that we do at the end of every workout. I also included a 10-minute resistance workout and 10-minute cardio workout in the back. Check them out if you haven't yet.

6
The Pizza Diet

How much Pizza does it take to get all your vitamins and minerals?

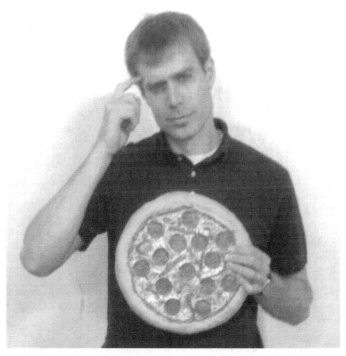

Assuming that there are small amounts of every vitamin and mineral in this pizza with meat and veggies (there are) How much pizza would you have to eat to hit your daily recommendations for all of the essential and known vitamins and minerals?

3.5 pizzas!!!

That's over 6500 Calories of Pizza!

This doesn't sound like a good idea! That's 3x the calories many of us need on a daily basis! We would be quite over weight. Most of us aren't going to hit that level of Calories from pizza like foods, but we might eat 3000 Calories of Pizza like food. Pizza like = High in calories and low in nutrients per calorie. If we eat 3000 Calories of pizza and our bodies require 6500 to get all the vitamins and minerals **it is quite possible for us to be GAINING weight and be malnourished.** Part of our cravings come from our body telling us to get more essential vitamins and minerals. Our body doesn't care how heavy we are as much as it cares if we are getting the essential ingredients for survival. If we can get those at a lower Calorie level our cravings may stop and we will be in a weight loss Calorie level!

Q: This sounds good. Weight loss without as much cravings? Where do I sign-up?

A: The produce section of the grocery store is where you sign-up. :o)

One of the targets we use for our clients is 1 pound of cooked and 1 pound of raw vegetables per day. (taken in part from Dr. Joel Fuhrman) If you have never eaten a vegetable before in your life I don't recommend you start at this level. Another one of our principles that I hope to over state is to strive to be better NOT PERFECT. So try to get closer to this number.

My motivation:
Cancer scares the crap out of me. I hate it. I know we live in a toxic world and that increases my chances of getting Cancer. I also know that Vegetables have proven themselves to decrease cancer risks

and increase life expectancy. So not just living longer but living healthier. I want to be active in my 80's not falling apart in a nursing home or already gone. Knowing the power of vegetables I have a choice to consciously eat more of them and stack the deck in my favor or ignore it and fail to do a simple thing that could affect the length and enjoyment of my life. I'm choosing veggies, but I ain't perfect. I don't hit it every day, but I'm better than before.

Prove It!

So I'm not much for taking anyone's word for things. I like to test them in my own way. We have a nutrition program that we use called Vitabot. I have decided it's better than other options for food journaling because it will allow you to see how healthy you are eating. It not only tracks major nutrients like FAT, SALT, CARBS, PROTEIN it also keeps track of many of our vitamins and minerals. It even gives you grades based on how you are doing.

I decided IF this 1 pound of cooked and 1 pound of raw recommendation was right that I should be able to eat a bunch of junk with the rest of my calories for the day and I should still score ok. So I added 1 pound of cooked Broccoli (454g) and 1 pound of fresh romaine lettuce (454g). Then to add my junk in I chose one of the most popular high calorie foods on the planet that's right…PIZZA! Of course pizza! This is the pizza diet section after all! So I needed to come up with an amount. I thought well I had a 1 pound of cooked veggies 1 pound of raw veggies how about 1 pound of pizza to start off with. I was blown away…it actually worked! The GPA was 3.31 out of 4.0 very respectable. And the overall calories for the day were only 1376 with 1168 of them coming from pizza! So there was only 208 Calories from vegetables but amazing benefits in such few Calories even if the rest of the day wasn't perfect.

I think this is a huge point. **WE DON'T HAVE TO BE PERFECT!** We just have to do pretty good on a couple things. So what if you had a slice of pizza, cookie, or cake. How that plays out with the rest of your food that day is a big factor. If you get enough veggies in you'll be sitting in a pretty good place, maybe even an awesome place!

So now measure your veggies for a couple days. Measure in grams and see how close you get to the 908g recommendation = 2 pounds. Most people think they eat a lot of vegetables until they actually keep track. Give it a shot and risk learning something new about yourself!

Note: If you want to do this right I want to help. I can give you a free 1-week trial of our food journaling software so you can see how this can work and get a big boost. Contact us at www.talltrainer.com/31lessonsbook

7
The Balance Illusion

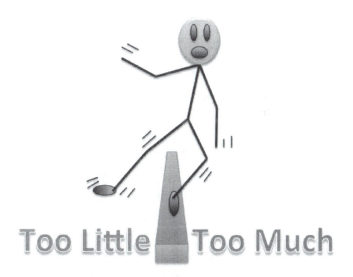

We all want "balance" in our lives. Balance in our work and family time. We strive to maintain a healthy weight and balance hard work with relaxation. We know automatically that extremes in most areas aren't healthy. All work and no play = unhealthy. Obesity is unhealthy and so is anorexia. So we quest after the elusive balance point. Somewhere between obesity and anorexia is a perfect balance point of the ideal weight.

We want to get to this balance point and stay there forever. For weight loss some of us have found this point and we felt "this is a good spot." I know more people

37

however that have never lived a day feeling like they found it. Many of our female clients will have the kind of body many women are wishing for and still they want to lose 5 more pounds. Others have reached a weight they have gotten to a half dozen times but each time they get there they hold for a short time and then put all the weight back on. They know how to lose weight but they don't know how to maintain. To find balance.

I think this lack of finding balance in our lives is due to the fact that we are viewing balance the wrong way. We are shooting for the impossible. At least in this life!

What is "balance" really?

The best picture I can give you for balance is one of the most extreme examples. The balance beam. It's an event in gymnastics that has balance as its main goal. These little gymnasts train years to be able to balance better than anyone else in the world. If you have watched the Olympics you've seen them do flips and land on this narrow beam! It's amazing! What I learned from them is that as they move they are constantly adjusting their balance. They do it with such small movements that to us non-balance world champions they look like they don't even have to try. Balance is the tiny microscopic point that exists between two extremes. No one ever gets stuck there!!!

What balance beam teaches us about life…

As my balance improves my fluctuations get smaller but they are still there. If I were to get on the balance beam I might be able to walk across it. I would probably be waving my hands and arms around like a maniac to not fall to either side. With practice my movements would get smaller but I would still have them just like the Olympians

7 – The Balance Illusion

do. So for weight loss/gain we might have lost 70 pounds and gained back 40. We then lose 40 and gain back 20. We lose 20 and gain back 10. This is what success often looks like. Eventually we get to a place that we stay in more like a 5-pound range. We aren't making progress when we lose 70 pounds and gain back 80, which happens too often. We don't catch it sooner. We wait until it's worse than ever before the alarms go off. It's not about whether or not you lose your balance. You will lose your balance. The key is how quickly you catch it again.

The biggest challenge in correcting balance is not OVER correcting and falling too far the other way. I have clients stand on a ½ ball called a Bosu to teach them about balance. Their first time on it seems inevitable that when they lose their balance one way they tend to overcorrect and send themselves falling off the other side. We do this in life too. Maybe we work too much and our family needs more urgent attention so we cut way back on work but we cut too far that work now becomes critical and we have to ditch family for a moment to put out a fire at work. The worst is getting stuck in this massive back and forth wobble. There will be seasons where you will be purposely out of balance to one side or the other. When you begin shifting back make sure you don't over do the shift an end up with the same problem again.

If I lose focus even if I'm well practiced at balance I am more likely to fall. This is over confidence or distraction.

Overconfidence - The saying "pride comes before a fall," applies here. (Proverbs 16:18) I get too prideful that I no longer need anyone's help or I don't even have to try. Typically a nasty wipe out is coming soon. Stay humble. Stay focused.

Fitness in Real Life

<u>Distraction is the other issue</u> - Something will come up. This is "life" after all. It's messy, not neat and tidy. It could be the death of a loved one, relationship issues, losing your job, car accident, etc. These things happen and they often come out of the blue. You would have to be a robot to not let these things effect your balance. You will get blindsided. Life is more like American Gladiators than the Olympics. Instead of peacefully flipping over a balance beam there is a huge force (gladiator) trying to knock you down! So it becomes not as important to maintain your balance as it is to get up sooner when you get knocked off.

There is a decision moment that happens when life knocks you on your back. You can stay there or get back up. I need you to know that you don't have to get back up instantly. We need to allow ourselves to grieve these moments too. But there comes a time when you need to grieve AND move. Also, you don't have to get up all by yourself. This is a decidedly American and mostly a Hollywood concept. You aren't weak if you get help from family, friends, and professionals. This is what a fulfilling life is all about, helping each other through the ups and downs. It is always an honor and so fulfilling when someone allows you to help them up.

When you don't have the strength to get up and try again, let someone help you, and ask God to help you!

8

Drink Water... Turn the Filter On

½ of your Weight in OZ of Water

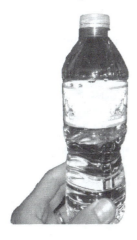

150 pound person should consume at least 75 oz. of water per day.

To give you an idea:
- There are 128 oz. in a gallon.
- 8 x 8 oz. glasses of water = 64 oz.
- Most plastic water bottles are 16.9 oz. X 5 = 84 ½ oz.

I learned a valuable lesson about hydration from our pool. We had a pool growing up. It was fun. I remember running across the stony driveway to jump in, play for hours, dry off to do it again the next day. So when the house we were buying had a pool I thought. Wow this is cool! Ok, I never had to keep a pool going as a kid (thanks Dad). It's a lot of work! Well I wasn't sure how much to run the filter so I ran it as little as possible. The water was cloudy all summer. I kept trying to vacuum and balance chemicals and it was still cloudy. The next year I decided to run the pump and filter like crazy. Walla, a crystal clear pool!

Then it struck me...the filter of our bodies are our kidneys.

The only way to turn on this filter is to drink water. Without that our bodies will look like a gunky pool on the inside. When I drink water I picture my body like a crystal clear pool. And this isn't much of an exaggeration.

How the kidneys work.

Diffusion - The process where molecules spread out across space naturally from an area of high concentration to low concentration. This means the kidneys don't pull stuff out of our blood, they allow stuff to diffuse out. This means to have clean blood we need to send a lot of liquid through them to get rid of the gunk of everyday life.

This is why you need to drink ½ your body weight in OZ of water. If you are _____ you need to drink more water than this.
- Sweating more
- In a hot environment
- Drinking coffee and alcohol
- Eating excessively dry food (more grains than veggies)

This is a massively powerful habit to master. If you can get this one going you will feel better in so many ways. You know what I hear from 90% of the people I mention this to? **"I drink a lot of water."** It seems everyone drinks plenty of water but why is it that the average person is chronically dehydrated? What is a lot? Have you ever kept track?

8 – Drink Water...Turn the Filter On

I have found that with desirable habits we do less than we think and certainly less than we want people around us to think (especially our personal trainer). And with non-desirable habits we do them more than we want to believe.

What's the big deal? Why do I need to drink water?

Issues related to not enough water:
- Constipation
- Arthritis
- High Blood
- High Cholesterol
- Excess Weight
- Low Energy
- Mid-Day Sleepiness
- Back and Neck Pain
- Stress
- Depression
- Asthma
- Allergies
- Headaches
- Etc…

Everything runs on water so its absence or shortage causes just about every function of the body to be worse. You can even find links to heart disease and cancer! Also, we come across toxins in our food, air, cleaning products, and pretty much everything around us. Our first level of defense is to rinse it out with water. We can lower our bodys toxic buildup first by simply drinking more water!

If you want to know more about how simple water can cure many issues you might be dealing with visit www.watercure.com and/or read Dr. F. Batmanghelidj book titled "Your Bodies Many Cries for WATER."

"We should first exclude the simpler cause for disease emergence in the body and then think of the more complicated."

"You're not sick; You're thirsty. Don't treat thirst with medication."

Dr. F. Batmanghelidj

I am personally thankful to Dr. Batmanghelidj for dedicating his career to the study of something with such little financial gain for himself. There is so much health we can gain from this simple "cure."

I have personally seen clients pick up the water habit and migraine headaches go away, blood pressure drops, and they feel SO MUCH BETTER! Blood pressure is a funny one because water helps remove excess salt from the body so instead of a low salt diet more of us probably need a high water diet!

Ok…now let's pretend I sold you on drinking more water. The next challenge you face is HOW?

Here are some tips to help you drink more of that amazing water:

- Drink water **1st thing in the morning** (aim for 20 oz) You've spent the night dehydrating. Getting up to pee and breathing both cause water loss and you probably did both during the night. The morning is your most dehydrated time of the day. This is why headaches, hangovers, and morning sickness have so much strength in the AM.

- Drink water **at every meal**. Or even better about 20 minutes BEFORE every meal. It will help make sure you don't over eat because you are thirsty.

- **Keep a water bottle handy**. If it's closer to you and more convenient you will drink more of it. Just like people sitting at a bar drink more alcohol than people sitting at a table away from the bar. Keep water close and you will drink more of it!

- **Keep water at your desk**. You work there a lot. You might spend nearly 8 hours+ straight in that seat if you brought your lunch and don't have a meeting. Drink water so you aren't so dead after work. The bathroom trips will help you stretch your legs and rest your eyes preventing issues with your back and knees and eyesight. That's a good deal!

- **Scheduled Chugging** can help you if you are REALLY out of the habit or really dedicated to making sure this happens. Pick some target times and amounts of water to have completed. Set an alarm on your phone to remind you it's time to finish that 20 ounces of water if you haven't already. First thing in the morning is a great time for this and maybe 10 am and 2 pm (before you get that afternoon tiredness). Don't do it before bed or you might disrupt your sleep more than normal.

- **Go 1 for 1 with coffee or alcohol**. If you have a cup of coffee have an extra glass of water. If you are hanging out, drink a glass of water for every alcoholic drink. It will help you keep calories low and make sure you aren't "that guy "or "that girl" at the party. Both coffee and alcohol cause us to pee more liquid than we are consuming. They might dehydrate us more than if we didn't have anything!

- **Pour glasses out of a gallon** so you know how much you've had. Fill a gallon jug with how much water you need to drink for the day and pour water from that into your drinking glass or water bottle. This way you KNOW you drank enough!

- **Try some rubber bands** or hair ties on your water bottle. Every time you finish it and refill it that day you move a band from the bottom to the top. When all the bands are at the top you finished your water!

Please give water a try. It's worth 3-4 days of focus to test and see how much you really are drinking on a regular basis. You just might feel fantastic! At the very least you'll get out of your chair more as you go to the bathroom!

9
Goal Setting

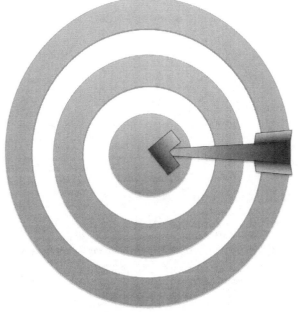

Do you achieve the goals you set for yourself?
Or
Are your Goals more like wishes that never come true?

If you answered yes to the first sentence then skip this section. You could probably write a better section than me on Goals. There are a couple main concepts that I want to make sure you understand about goals.

- SMART Goals
- Process vs. Outcome Goals
- Shrink the Change
- Review Time

Everyone seems to start with **SMART goals** and your goals do need to hit these requirements to be helpful:

Specific – Not general or vague "feel better" or "lose weight"
Measureable – You need to be able to tell you hit it with real data
Actionable – Something you can do something about
Realistic – Making a million dollars next week (is everything but realistic)
Time – It has a due date

Once you have those ideas down it stops you from making goals that you look back on and say "I can't tell if I did it!"

Process vs. Outcome

I think we need both of these types of goals. They play off each other well to help us actually get where we are trying to go! Most people think outcome when it comes to goals. I want to get more sleep. I want to lose 5 pounds. (Both aren't SMART goals by the way). I see the main purpose of an outcome goal is to be the carrot.

When talking about getting something to happen motivation is often talked about in terms of carrots and sticks. When thinking of trying to get a stubborn donkey moving you can lead it with a carrot or whack it with a stick. Working on getting something or working on avoiding something. It is my experience that carrots (positive motivation) work better than sticks (negative motivation) for lasting change.

You need something to get excited about! The outcome goal is that excitement. The Process Goal is what it takes to get there on a daily basis. The outcome might be to lose 5 pounds this month or to be able to button your favorite jeans at the end of the month. Whatever it is, it needs to feel exciting to reach it! It's that excitement that gets you through some of the challenges of the day to day achievement of the goal.

The process goal may look something like this. I will drink 16 oz of water within one hour of waking 5 days per week. I will eat over 10 grams of protein for breakfast 5 days per week. (See Craving Management section in the back for goal ideas and the habit section on how to make sure you have a new habit setup properly).

The process goals are the steps it will take daily to reach the outcome by the deadline. Most things we set outcome goals for take several consistent steps to achieve.

"A goal without a plan is just a wish." - Jeremy

People set these wishes in our fitness program all the time. We set goals every month and sometimes people will say, "I want to lose 5 pounds this month." The only problem is they don't have a plan to do anything different this month compared to last month. It has a slight feeling of hoping a weight loss fairy will stop by and grant your wish. Please don't wait for the fairy (I'm mostly sure they don't exist).

Shrink the Change

The other problem I see is a type of impatience that kills our momentum. If we are in the habit of setting BIG goals but not achieving them we start to believe goal setting is a waste of time. Sometimes people will be tempted to bring their unachieved goal from last month into the next month. I would encourage you not to do this. Make it fresh and make it smaller. We do not expect our children to go from crawling to Olympics in one day, but we do go from no achievement to aiming for super achievement.

If you follow successful people you will see that they gradually built up their goal achieving. If you want to lose 10 pounds and you lost zero last month while you were trying to lose 10 maybe lower it to 5 pounds or 3 pounds or even 1 pound. Depending on your track record with goals you might need to start super easy. In the book "Switch: How to Change Things When Change is Hard" by Chip and Dan Heath one of the points they talk about is growing your perception of yourself and shrinking the change. If you grow your perception by achieving small goals and shrink the big goals down until you believe you can do it, you'll probably do it!

Which Goal Will Be Achieved?

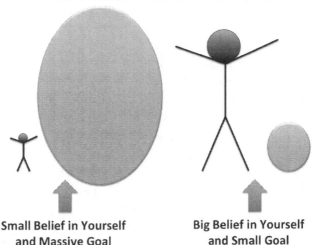

Small Belief in Yourself and Massive Goal

Big Belief in Yourself and Small Goal

One of my favorite examples of this shrinking a goal down is Linda (who's names been changed to protect the innocent). She had a goal to walk 3 miles every day. She walked only 2 times last month. So she set the goal to just put her shoes on and step outside everyday. It was a smaller goal, one that could fit into even the most crazy day. She stuck to the goal and even managed to go for a walk most times she stepped out (not all). Who would make more progress? Someone who sets an ambitious goal but never takes action, or someone who sets a smaller goal that they stick with?

We know the answer to that one.

Review Time

The most forgotten key to goals is to check up on them! Many people set a goal but don't set and plan a review time. The goal just fades away like a distant memory. When you are making your goals also make a plan for when you will review. If you want to up the likelihood of you actually getting there, you can ask someone for a coffee date on that day to ask you about your goals. You can up the stakes with this person by coming up with incentives or consequences if needed. Remember that incentives and consequences are best for short-term goals. Hopefully if you are making your goals right there are intrinsic positive effects of achieving your goals so you don't need carrots or sticks as much.

That's enough talk about goals. Now write some SMART process and outcome goals and plan a review time!

10
The Crabs
(Why People Pull You Down)

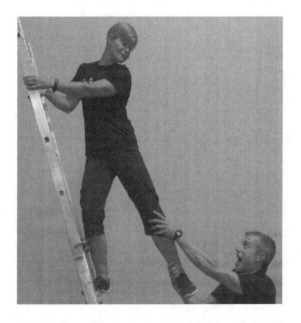

Time to get real... (I'm not always this big of a jerk)

When Sarah and I first got married we started working out together. In my mind I was the "Personal Trainer" and I was the "MAN" so I figured I should be better at all things physical. When she started beating me I started discounting her performance. Either her technique was off so that made it easier on her or she wasn't using enough weight that's why she got done first. Basically I

10 – The Crabs (why people pull you down)

was being a jerk. I didn't realize how much my ego was wrapped up in this and how I was slashing her down to protect myself.

I call these people crabs because crabs are self-policing. You can put crabs in a bucket with the top off and when one starts to climb out others will actually grab it and pull it back down. It is unfortunate that people do this too. (even me)

I dare you to lose 10 lbs, 20 lbs., or more and begin getting close to your goal weight without getting some negative reactions from some people around you. (Some of us may have had these reactions ourselves about someone else without knowing why we were reacting so negatively)

Why would someone say something negative about someone doing something positive? When someone steps out and accomplishes something awesome there are two choices we have in our reaction.

- Discount their achievement so we don't feel uncomfortable anymore about ourselves.
- Be inspired by them and begin taking steps in a positive direction.

Unfortunately many people feel hopeless so they instantly, and unconsciously, turn to negativity.

"You don't need to lose weight"
"You're too skinny"
Translation: If you need to lose weight then I REALLY need to lose weight.

"That's way too much work for me."
Translation: I don't believe in myself enough to try right now.

"Come on have a (cookie, pizza, or other treat). You can't have any fun now that you're on a diet?"
Translation: If you eat with me I won't feel like a pig eating this while you stand strong.

"Yes, you did better than me but your form wasn't as good as mine."
Translation: I'm not grown up enough to encourage someone for doing a better job than me because my ego is too fragile. :o)

Important note: find people who don't project their feelings onto you and get their feedback. You do need to hear if there is something you might be doing wrong, but you'll hear it in the style of delivery (delivering the truth with love).

How do we deal with this?
- You might limit your interactions with this person if possible. (I'm glad Sarah didn't choose this one! Though we didn't workout as often until I began choosing option number 2 above)
- Get time with positive people too. People who have climbed farther out of the bucket and can lift you and inspire you to their level.
- Understand that for most of these negative people their reaction is unconscious. They are often not conscious that they are being a jerk. (like I was)
- Ask them why they keep discounting your hard work. (They will not have an answer right then and might get defensive but they might take time to think about it later. This is what Sarah did for me.)
- Explain to them your reason why (if you feel strong enough for a possible jerky response) –

10 – The Crabs (why people pull you down)

> Your hurt and struggle will help them see that you aren't doing this because you want them to feel bad but because you need to feel better.

- If it's your spouse – go to counseling. Sarah and I go often :o)
- I guess this shouldn't be last but I don't want you to think this book is only for Christians…Pray to God for that person and for courage for yourself. It will help (or more accurately He will help).

This negativity can be crushing to some of our clients weight loss efforts. Stay strong. Speak up for your feelings (and do it with love).

Also, check out the section about stress management and the book "Boundaries" by Henry Cloud.

11

The Laws of Science and Your Metabolism

"The **law of conservation of mass** or **principle of mass conservation** states that for any system closed to all transfers of matter and energy, the mass of the system must remain constant over time, as system mass cannot change quantity if it is not added or removed. Hence, the quantity of mass is "conserved" over time. The law implies that mass can neither be created nor destroyed, although it may be rearranged in space."

"First law of thermodynamics: When energy passes, as work, as heat, or with matter, into or out from a system, its internal energy changes in accord with the law of conservation of energy."

Thank you Wikipedia.com!

So what?...

So…Bad news. You almost certainly don't have a slow metabolism.

FAT is made out of Carbon, Hydrogen, and Oxygen. Those things don't disappear into energy. The energy comes from breaking the bonds between those elements but the elements continue to exist and they still weigh something.

So where do they go?

$$C_{55}H_{104}O_6 + 78O_2 \longrightarrow 55CO_2 + 52 H_2O$$

FAT + Oxygen   **Carbon Dioxide + Water**

This is where the FAT Goes!...
84% of fat pounds are exhaled as CO_2
16% of fat pounds are excreted as H_2O

So…most fat leaves by breathing? That's some heavy air! We don't usually think of air as having weight to it but it certainly does! Like feeling how heavy a propane tank is on your outdoor grill to know if you've got enough in there to grill some chicken. :o)

If you stay alive, stand up, move around, or exercise it all takes energy. You cannot eat hardly anything and move a bunch and somehow avoid losing weight. This energy to move has to come from somewhere. If it's not coming from food it has to come from stored energy on your body.

Now if you cut back on your calorie intake you may notice a drop in your energy for the day. Our body will feel less energetic when underfed. That is a starvation protection mechanism. If you watch a survivalist type TV show you can see this really well. They take people and put them in an isolated location and they try to out survive each other. They are hardly getting any food so they are tired and irritable. When there isn't any specific task they have to do they are for the most part laying around. Their body is trying to save energy. If we cut our nutrition too far and not the right way we will find low energy and a slower weight loss than expected. But, it would still happen especially with exercise added in.

When exercise and "dieting" aren't working...

Most of the time when I come across someone who thinks they have a slow metabolism they are not keeping close track of what they are eating. They will be exercising and saying they are eating at the lowest recommended level of 1200 Calories (or lower!) but they won't be losing weight. The math doesn't work out. It doesn't pass the laws of thermodynamics. They are eating more than they say or possibly more than they even know!

I encourage them to become a Calorie detective to search out where they are coming from. I have found that it's typically one or more of these 3 places:

- **They are not measuring their food** so they don't know how much they are actually eating. This can easily make someone's estimates about 40%-100% off. Meaning they have possibly eaten twice as many calories as they think. It's like thinking you ate 1200 Calories when really it was 2400.

- **They forgot some food they ate**. They ate and either they planned to write it down later or their brain wasn't even invited. They ate without realizing they were eating. This forgotten food is enough to make you think you have a slow metabolism because it seems like you hardly eat.

- **They are embarrassed of their eating habits** and either they are trying to hide it from others (trainer included) or they even block it out themselves. They feel so guilty of the sleeve of oreos they just polished off that they pretend it didn't happen.

The first two can be fixed by keeping a food journal. Over time you begin catching yourself in eating moments thinking "I haven't measured this yet!" You also get better at measuring and you begin to realize how EASY calories are to eat! The third point is much harder and might involve time with a counselor to beat that one. Some of our other sections deal with the emotional eating component a little more.

I would say about 80% of my clients who claim to have a slow metabolism actually have a problem in those 3 places. For the other 20% the problem may be related to the need for Carb-Cycling (read: "I overate…why is my weight down" section) or they have actually started moving significantly less during their non-workout times of the day.

When you are tempted to shift the blame onto your metabolism please consider the laws of thermodynamics. On top of this, consider the consequences of passing the buck and blaming your metabolism. If you blame metabolism, height, age, kids schedules, or any other factor that you feel no ability to control you are essentially giving up on yourself. "It's not my fault it's _____." Even if you did have a slow metabolism there is no amount of slow that you can't do battle against.

Don't give up! If it's harder for you, so be it. You can still do it and it will be worth it!

12

There is no "I can't"

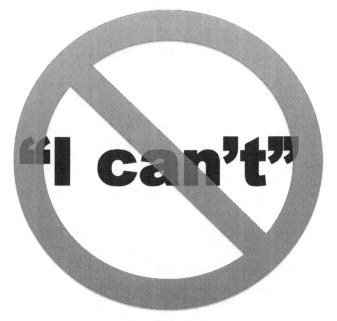

This has been a Tall Trainer Philosophy from the very beginning. It's roots are in the Bible, Philippians 4:13 "I can do all things through Christ who strengthens me." The "I Can't" phrase comes out of our mouth far too often. Every time it does we give away some of our personal power, control, and choice. Probably the most common example that I catch myself using this sometimes still is when someone invites you to an event and you have a conflict already on your calendar. We say "sorry I can't come." In this context we are trying to make it seem like we are powerless to change the schedule so we aren't saying no to someone. The truth is we can. We are choosing not to. It would be more true to say "I'm sorry I have already committed to another event at that time and I want to honor my commitment." (That flows pretty natural right? Ok, maybe not.)

Now you don't have to go out and change the way you say everything over night. But I want you to be aware when you are making yourself powerless. I saw this come up so often training people that the words "there is no 'I can't'" were on the walls of my first fitness studio.

We say "I can't" when the truth is…
…We don't want to
…It's going to be hard
…We aren't sure if we can

I find people get stuck in their weight loss, finances, job, etc. because of this very habit of creating powerlessness. I hear this phrase come out most often when someone has completed 12 great repetitions of an exercise and I say, "just 3 more!" When we are tired and have low belief in ourselves it's tempting to throw an "I can't" out there so we don't have to try. If we try we might fail and failure is scary to so many. (Except to those who are successful because they failed many times trying to get to where they are.) A fun activity to ask when you find yourself spitting an "I can't" out of your mouth is to follow it up with a "what if I can?" What if I can do those last 3 repetitions? What if I can lose those last 10 pounds that I always struggle with? What if I can…? The thoughts that pop into your head are a lot more interesting after a question like that than a boring brain halting "I can't". Another break through question is "how can I?" When we ask good questions we often get good answers, even when we are asking ourselves.

Fitness in Real Life

We need to not only be on guard for our own limiting beliefs but also the limiting beliefs of others. One "you can't" type comment from a certain person at a certain moment can be all it takes to stop us from pursuing our dreams.

I still remember when I was planning to move back to my hometown after learning the personal training field in Texas. I had encouraged my Mom to get a trainer at a local gym to look out for her posture. I told her what to look for in a trainer and she found one who also taught classes at the local community college. When she told him what I planned on doing he abruptly told her, "you can't make a living as a personal trainer here!" He was putting his "I can't" on ME! Well I knew better and had been trained by some of the best so I made the jump. It was challenging and for a year I lived with my parents to get the business started but since then I have enjoyed 9 years of supporting myself and my family as a personal trainer. I think I CAN!

"If you think you can do a thing or think you can't do a thing, you're right." - Henry Ford

If you get this thinking right there is not much that will stop you from getting to your goal. If you get it wrong just about anything can stop you.

A dash of realism: There are limits in this world some that are foolish to challenge. I don't need to try to get on the Men's Olympic Gymnast team. I'm 6'3" and well past the 18-20 year old prime gymnast age and I have a ruptured disc in my lower back. I won't say "I can't" but there may be a better use of my time, a job and purpose that God has called me and created me to perform. So I often make sure to remind people as we are shooting for the stars in our physical fitness that we can just add an "Is this wise?", after our "no I can't" declaration. This helps to make sure we are making a quality decision. I can try to make the Olympic Gymnastic team but is it wise?

The people I see become successful seem to have a more childlike approach to their goals. If you ask a kid if they can dance they will show you they can right there. If you ask if they can play the piano they say YES. And if you ask them if they can touch the moon they try to jump!

So my question to you as you have those excuses and limitations bouncing around in your head...What if you CAN?

13
Am I Gaining Muscle?

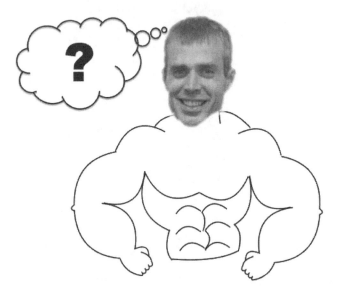

When the scale doesn't move and we've been exercising and watching what we eat this is one of the first questions we ask. It's a good question because you can be the same weight and look very different based on WHAT your body is made of. If we have 10 pounds of extra fat or 10 pounds of extra muscle there is a BIG difference in how we look and how we feel.

How to know if you are gaining muscle when the scale doesn't move...

- Your % Body Fat goes down
- Your waist circumference goes down

13 – Am I Gaining Muscle?

- Your pants fit better (at the waist at least)

If you don't see some change in at least one of those areas you need to assume you are stuck vs. gaining muscle. Now you need to give it a couple weeks before you decide you're stuck. But at the 2-week mark if you can't see changes you can probably review your habits and tweak them to get more and faster results.

It happens often that some trainers will tell their clients they are gaining muscle even without any measurement that confirms it. That it is done usually to try to keep a client with weak motivation from quitting before they get the results. I understand why this is done but I also know that it can delay positive change if we are moving in the wrong direction. Truthfully a trainer can put you through the perfect workouts 6 days a week (rest the 7th) and the best meal plan ever but there is still so much of the success that rides on what you do outside of workouts. You actually have to follow through on the nutrition.

Just in case you are reading this section and wondering why anyone would want to ask "Am I gaining muscle?" Here is a couple points on why you would want to build muscle.

- A pound of muscle burns 6-10 Calories at rest/day (10 pounds = 60-100 Cals/day!) You get to eat more!
- You gain strength too. Loss of muscle and strength is a serious issue as we age making us more frail and leading us to be more dependent on others.
- Muscle hides in all the right places making your figure more ideal, while fat hangs on the worst places making us look worse.

- A feeling of strength is empowering and can increase confidence in every area of our lives.
- For the women who think they are going to look gross with muscle we aren't talking that much muscle. It will give you definition in your arms and shape to your legs. Thankfully this lift weight get huge myth has been mostly culturally debunked.

How to build muscle

There are a million different theories on how to gain muscle. There is the science way, there is the gym science way, there are ways popular in sports, other cultures, and on and on. Instead of making this confusing which is super easy to do, I want to make this simple. I have found a common theme running through all these theories.

1. Work the muscle to it's limit…and beyond sometimes
2. Eat enough protein to build it back

That's all it takes. It's a two-step process. Both steps are challenging in their own way. They both require consistency to see the benefit. Resistance Training Exercise needs to be done regularly and at a challenging intensity. And proper nutrition needs to be coming into the body constantly.

Mistakes in Exercise That Cost You Muscle

Too much cardio and not enough resistance training - Muscles never get the message you need more strength. **Too long of resistance training workouts** - 40 minutes is good, stress hormones build up after that.

13 – Am I Gaining Muscle?

Not getting the last reps - Stopping too soon sometimes people leave 5+ repetitions not done. This means they could have done significantly more work on the muscle.

Not Consistent - Workouts don't happen with regularity enough to build on each other.

Mistakes in Nutrition That Cost You Muscle

Not enough protein - Can't build more muscle without the building blocks

Too much sugar, bread, and junk - This food helps us gain fat not muscle, have for a treat.

Alcohol - It's an estrogenic compound which means it tells our bodies to store fat not build muscle. Beer belly isn't just a funny term!

For me personally the nutrition side is harder than the exercise. Getting that protein level is the key. If you hired someone to build you a brick house but didn't give them any bricks they wouldn't get very far would they? Our body works much the same way. It might actually deconstruct muscle in one part of the body to build it up in another harder used area. Eating enough protein allows the body to build new muscle from the amino acids in the protein.

The research points to .64 - .9 grams of protein per pound of body weight to build muscle. So a 150-pound person would need to take in 96g-135g of protein.

Tips on protein:
- If trying to go vegan you will probably need a protein powder for one or more of your meals.
- Chicken and fish are wonderful but so is grass fed beef.
- Lunch meats can be used for snacks

Fitness in Real Life

- You will get some protein from vegetables (and grains a little) so it doesn't have to be all meat
- Eggs in the morning are a great trick to get jump started – if you get behind on protein it can be tough to catch up! A whole egg is fine unless you find your Calories getting too high.
- If dairy isn't an issue for you, then Greek yogurt and cottage cheese can give you more variety for your protein and fit that "snack" type feeling.
- Protein without enough fat, water, and vegetables can constipate you. Have tons of water and vegetables and aim for fat to be about ½ the grams of protein. (if you are eating 100g protein then 50g of fat should be ok)

Basically, you are only gaining muscle if you are:
A.) Working the muscles hard – they will be sore sometimes (not all the time)
B.) Getting your protein in daily

If you aren't working on both of these things your weight maintenance (or gain) is not likely to signal a gain in muscle. I would be thrilled if more women especially would put a focus on gaining muscle and less on their scale weight. When I do see someone "get it" they feel less cravings and are more full during the day. They usually have better energy too. Remember gaining muscle is hard it won't happen without some attention. Give it a try for a week and see if you notice a difference.

IT'S TIME FOR MUSCLES!!! :o)

14

Are you living in a RAT TRAP? Or a RAT PARK?

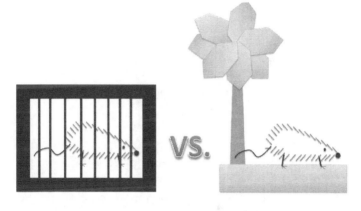

When soldiers were over in Vietnam they were under such difficult circumstances that many used powerful drugs to cope. Even by getting addicted to Heroin which is considered so addictive that once you are addicted you will never quit. When the soldiers came back it is no secret they didn't get a great greeting. While some sought continued comfort in drugs there were many that were able to stop permanently. Even on a heavily addictive substance.

It was this fact that got researchers to question how and why this was happening. The original experiments were on rats in a cage with an unlimited supply of self-injected heroin. It's not surprising that they kept injecting themselves until they died. The conclusion seemed to point to no hope of escaping addiction.

Along came researcher Bruce Alexander, he felt that the experiment was like shooting fish in a barrel. His hypothesis was that, "Severely distressed animals, like severely distressed people, will relieve their distress pharmacologically if they can." With no hope or even entertainment it made sense the rats chose the drugs. Bruce ran a different experiment. He created "Rat Park", a rat paradise with everything rats love. Both sexes so they can mate and raise a litter, balls to play with, running wheels, tunnels, lots of room to explore, places to dig, etc. In the Rat Park there was still the drug option. There were two water bottles one with sugar water laced with morphine and the other with just clean water. The Rats showed no signs of addiction.

That wasn't enough so he put rats in solitary confinement with only the drugged water as an option for 57 days to get them nice and addicted. When they were added back to Rat Park they shed their addictions even though they went through withdrawal!!!

What does this mean for us?...

There is no arguing that high calorie, especially high sugar (carbohydrate) foods trip the same pleasure centers of the brain that opiates like heroin and morphine hit. They have their own level of addiction. Some of our weight loss challenges stem from this addiction to these types of foods. So, how are we to cope? How do we shed this addiction?

Change your cage.

14 – Are you living in a RAT TRAP?

Unlike the Rats we live in a prison of our own design. We have more choices than we care to admit. If we choose to change our environment we may not NEED the pleasure these foods provide.

One of the many tips and activities from a book we recommend "The Four-Day Win" by Martha Beck is to try 3 things:

Write down your obstacles that are keeping you from having a Rat Park life, then choose to either:

Bag it – Let it go or get rid of it. There are some things that can be dropped. It may be hard to let go but it's possible. It might take some counseling.

Barter it – Trade it or delegate it. An example of my life is I delegate car repair to a mechanic. It stressed me out because I don't have experience or understanding in that area. Instead of trying to figure it out and be miserable I choose to pay someone to do something they are good at with the money I make doing something I'm good at.

Better it – Some things shouldn't be dropped altogether and shouldn't be given to someone else. These things need to be bettered. An example could be exercise. Dropping it doesn't maintain your health and someone else exercising for you doesn't help you either. You can find a way to make exercise more fun. Many people have found our program to be that solution for them. They don't like exercise but they have more fun in our creative, energetic, positive, and social environment.

Get out your notepad and start creating your own Human Park!

15
Spot Reduction

The removal of fat from one spot on the body by exercising that area…

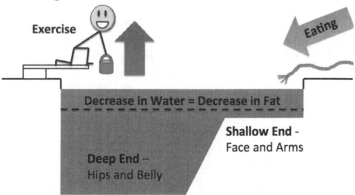

This one is explained best in a story:
I have a pool. It's nice. We love it in the summer. The outside temperature feels like it drops 15 degrees once you jump in the pool. And it came with the house, how lucky can you get?

Well this is a nice pool. It has stairs going into the shallow end and a deep end with a diving board (which I do flips off of) and a slide. It even has one of those lights underwater so you can light up the pool at night and feel like you are a movie star. It's a pretty awesome pool and I wouldn't change a thing about it. But, let's say I decided that there was one little thing that bugged me about the pool. The shallow end was perfect but I felt like the deep end was far too deep. I'm not much of a handy man but I like to work hard so I go and get a bucket and start scooping water out of the deep end and pouring it into the grass. I spend hours and hours scooping, carrying, and dumping water. ONLY in the deep end mind you, because the shallow end is perfect, I just want less water in the deep end.

I think we already know what would happen? Wouldn't the water level of the whole pool go down even though I only worked on the deep end? This is going to be a horribly traumatic statement I am about to make to many of you who have been tricked.

OUR BODIES WORK JUST LIKE THE POOL!!!!

Exercising one part of the body burns calories and removes fat from the whole body just like a bucket removes water from the whole pool.

Our belly and hips are obviously our deep end. They have far more fat storage than anywhere else. Our body is smart that way. It's the easiest place to carry extra weight. Could you imagine if we just gained extra weight in our hands? Everything we did would take so much work! Keeping the weight close to our center of gravity helps it to be more manageable.

Did you ever wonder why you notice weight loss in people's faces and arms first? It's because that is the shallow end! If you take a foot of water out of the pool you will certainly notice it most in the shallow end. In my pool you'd have a few stairs to go down before you even got to the water!

If you still don't believe our bodies work like that I want you to fully imagine the body allowing location specific weight loss based on exercise in that area. This means those guys doing 1,000 crunches a day but nothing else would have RIPPED six-pack abs and fat arms and faces. You've never seen it happen that way have you? I know I haven't. That's like taking water out of the pool and seeing a hole in the water where the bucket was. So glad it doesn't happen like that. It would be so hard to exercise and keep people looking balanced.

Don't do crunches for belly fat and arm exercises for back of the arm fat...

Trying to lose fat in these areas with these types of exercises is like bailing water out of the pool with a shot glass. AB and arm exercises are not the big calorie burners. Those exercise are still helpful but if we focus on totally body intense exercise, that's like pulling water out of the pool with a big ole garbage can! We'll have much better and faster results.

Extending the pool analogy – Why exercise alone doesn't work.

While we are on the pool analogy it can be a great place to talk about why exercise without proper nutrition doesn't work. Exercising is like the bucket pulling water out of the pool and nutrition is controlling the flow of the water hose. For us, both are happening everyday. If you eat a lot, the hose is turned on full throttle (maybe even a fire hose!). That's going to take a lot of bailing to even keep the water at the same level. Eventually you might tire out give up and the water level will rise. To get the most results from our fitness and weight loss program, we have to keep vital nutrients coming in without a surplus in calories. We need to burn those extra calories with our workouts and our metabolism boosting activities. Imagine how fast the water would evaporate if you could control how hot it was outside. Building muscle is like increasing evaporation on the pool. Without extra exercise (bailing) your body will burn more Calories at rest. High intensity interval training and resistance training also have a larger

15 – Spot Reduction

EPOC (Excess Post-exercise Oxygen Consumption). This means they cause metabolism to be elevated for minutes and hours after the workout depending on intensity. Some studies have witnessed this effect 24-48 hours after the workout!

So instead of spending our available time trying to spot reduce the butt, thighs, abs, or arms we need to use that time generating more muscle and a bigger after burn. It's also not a bad idea to figure out how to better regulate the inflow of food as well. If you don't, there is no way to out exercise a fire hose of food coming in daily. Exercise and nutrition…nutrition and exercise…for best results become better at both!

16

Your problem probably isn't where your injury is…

I need more people to understand this because understanding this concept is the key to freeing yourself from nagging aches and pain.

On the surface this doesn't make sense. If my back hurts I have a back problem. If my knee hurts I have a knee problem. Yes and No. Of course it is problematic to go about life with a hurt knee or back. I'm not trying to tell you that it isn't painful and draining.

BUT…the problem that **CAUSED** the pain is probably located somewhere else.

The best way I have found to explain this idea which sounds weird at first is thinking of the body like a factory assembly line. When everyone is doing their job well the factory output is high and things run smooth. However, if you are next to someone on the line and they aren't doing their job (or only part of it), now you have to do their job AND your job. You are working HARD! Which one of you do you think is going to complain first?

Assembly Line Effect

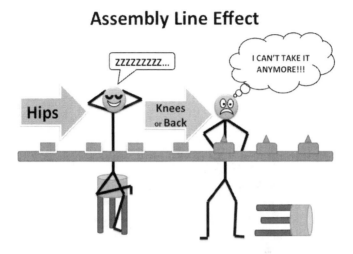

I'm going to guess that you will be the first to complain or just collapse. You weren't the problem but now you look like the problem if you are the worker out on workers compensation.

This can happen all over the body. The place I see it most is the hips, back, and knees. With our current lifestyles of all this sitting, our hips stop doing their job and the back and knees often pick up the slack. They sometimes can go years doing this without a complaint but eventually it get's too much and you start to have pain in the back and/or the knees.

People will get injections, knee replacements, back surgeries, pain medicine all to treat the symptoms of this pain and not the cause. Don't get me wrong there is a time and place for ALL those interventions, but it should come after a thorough investigation and assessment. A GREAT physical therapist will do this in the medical community. A great personal trainer might be able to help before it get's that far. An average therapist or trainer won't find this and will treat what you came in for and send you on your way.

Stability and Mobility Zones

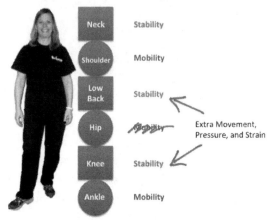

We have different needs in different parts (joints) of our body. Certain areas need stability while other areas need mobility. In the figure above you can see how these basically alternate through the body. Our problem lies in the fact that modern life has made most of our mobility zones less mobile, which then requires extra movement, pressure, and strain into our stability zones. Here are a few of the most common issues and were they come from.

- Less Mobility in the Hips -> More strain in Lower Back and Knees
- Less Mobility in Shoulder Girdle -> More Strain in Neck and Rotator Cuff (some Low Back)
- Less Mobility in Ankle -> More Strain on Knees

To fix these Mobility issues takes some focus. If you are not being protective of your stability zones while you exercise and stretch your mobility zones you will continue to injure your knees, back, neck, and rotator cuff.

Priorities to Protect Stability Zones and Stretch Mobility Zones Safely:

1.) Posture

A great exercise done with bad posture is a bad exercise. We do not get the full benefit and could be building an injury. Above all work to have great posture at all times. When we have great posture the areas that are tight get loosened and the areas that are weak get strengthened in the right proportion. It makes you weaker initially to hold good posture. You will use less weight and have to move slower. If you can be patient and check your ego at the door you will build a strong and great feeling body.

2.) Range of Motion

If a large range of motion causes you to lose posture you need to narrow the range of motion to an amount you can control. You can try to increase this range of motion by challenging the limits of flexibility and strength at that area as long as doing so doesn't cause you to break posture. Posture is more important than range of motion, but a full range of motion will provide additional strength and ability.

3.) Resistance

Resistance could be adding additional weight, time, speed, or complexity. Basically resistance can be anything that makes it harder. What happens often is people increase the weight they are lifting so much that they start lifting with improper posture and poor range of motion. Lifting at the most challenging resistance level is important to send the "time to get stronger" message to the muscles. If this is done while sacrificing the first two priorities it ain't worth it. The sacrifice will more likely damage joints and lead to injury and not health or strength.

Other considerations when dealing with pain:
Proper Stretching and Resistance Training Exercises for Hips, Ankles, and Shoulder Blades will begin to provide relief. Don't take painkillers before a workout unless required by your doctor because you need to STOP ASAP when you feel pain. Pain during a workout is usually more painful later. If the painkiller masks too much of the pain you will overdo it and probably have a rough day and poor sleep.

Acceptable Pain and Bad Pain During Exercise

	Feeling	Location	Duration
Acceptable	Gradual Warming or Burning type Sensation	• Large Area • Away from joints	Burning gone as soon as you stop or within a minute Muscle soreness for < 3 days
Bad	Sharp, shooting, stabbing, grinding or Sudden Onset	• Specific Area • Small Area - Often can be covered by a thumb • In or around the joints	Still hurts after minutes of rest Soreness lasting longer than 4 days

* Stop exercise immediately if you feel any "bad" signs and consult a professional.
** If you are unsure of the "acceptable" signs see a professional also. When in doubt use caution.

This would take too long to describe here but if you are interested in a basic workout and stretches that can fit most people you can look at the appendix in the back of this book. (Depending on the severity of your injury/issue you may need one on one attention or guidance in a highly structured group environment like our fitness boot camp)

Final word on this:

It is possible that your problem has started with tight hips and caused knee pain and it has gone unchanged for too long that the damage to your knees is irreversible. In this situation you might have "BAD" knees, BUT you can **manage** the pain better by putting the right exercises for mobility and strength into your daily routine. Get started on this ASAP because the longer you go in pain the harder the solution becomes.

17

Is your environment making you fatter?

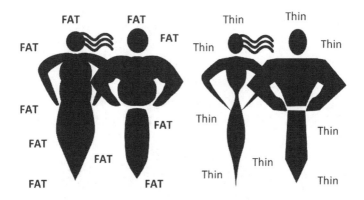

Yes!

I'm all about accepting personal responsibility for our health and our life, BUT your environment can be part of your struggle to lose weight or keep weight off. Personal responsibility comes in once we are aware of this issue then we have a responsibility to do something about our environment. We have a lot more choice than we think.

Why I beg Sarah not to bake…

I do not have some sort of great self-control or willpower that most people would assume a personal trainer with abs has. If there are cookies on the counter under that plastic wrap I will eat at least 6 per day (1/2 a cookie at a time). At about 100 Calories or more per cookie I'm looking at a bonus 600+ Calories for the day. If we had cookies in the house everyday I would probably gain 60 pounds in a year! (Thankfully I don't have to beg Sarah much since we are on the same page on this.)

If I didn't setup my environment to make healthy eating more brainless I would easily be holding 30+ pounds of FAT right now. This is not an uncommon reaction to visible food. Food and behavior researcher Brian Wansink, Ph.D. of Cornell studies how we interact with food. They have some awesome and eye opening studies that he has published in both of his books "Mindless Eating" and "Slim by Design." If you want to get a PhD in understanding your food environment I recommend you read his books! There is no way I can cover everything in this short section. He found that if there is visible cereal in the kitchen when you walk in that the people in that house weigh 20 pounds more than people without visible cereal. Wow! 20 pounds!

So knowing this we can begin to turn a fattening environment into a skinny making environment.

Things I would try to do:

- Shop off a list at the grocery store and be full when you are shopping and you will buy less sugary carbohydrates. If it gets in your cart it gets in your house if it gets in your house it will be in you! If you cannot be trusted at the store send someone else!
- Put healthy foods like fruits or veggies on the counter or eye level in the fridge. The crisper is where veggies go to die! We told our classes about

this one and we had a husband wife duo in class. When he got home his beer was in the vegetable crisper! That's environmental design!

- Put unhealthy foods as far away as possible. Make it tough to get to them and in a place you don't look often. One client I had loved ice cream and instead of saying no or never we said just go "out" for ice cream. They didn't go every night like they used to when the ice cream was in the freezer.

- If you buy in bulk, separate it into small baggies as soon as possible. If you eat out of the big package you'll eat more. People that buy in bulk tend to eat that food faster. It's like the toilet paper roll. When it's BIG you use more but when it's running low you take a smaller amount (don't pretend like you don't do this too!)

- Eat off of smaller plates. It sounds goofy but the research proves it time and time again. I'd make sure you didn't have anything over a 10' plate to eat off of. We like our plates to be ¾ full so if it's smaller you will eat less without even thinking about it. Sure it's only going to factor in at about 10% but that's big time over the course of a year! www.smallplatemovement.org.

- Make smaller dinners so you don't have as much extra. Or at least prepare less starchy carbs. You can make too much protein and veggies and eating a little more broccoli is not very likely to be your weight loss nemesis.

There are about as many ideas to make your environment skinny friendly as there are people. **Just sit and think about making good choices easier and bad choices harder and you'll come up with a bunch.** The trick then is actually setting up your environment. Knowing

17 – Is your environment making you fatter?

small plates is a good idea does nothing for you until you garage sale your platters and buy some nice small plates.

We don't stop eating when we are full.

This is an important concept to agree with. Thankfully there is research to support it so if you disagree you are just being disagreeable. Many of us were taught to clean our plate. For some of us throwing out a bite of food could cause Post Traumatic Stress. Think of those starving kids in _____. I think parental pressure factors in here for some of us but I think mindlessness is the bigger factor. Have you ever opened a bag of chips and sat on the couch only to find that after an hour you are dumping the last crumbs into your mouth going "Oh man I can't believe I ate them all!" The signal to stop was the bag getting to the bottom. The problem is if the bag is 1000-1500 Calories you are very unlikely to lose weight in the near future. Set up your environment to tell you to stop eating sooner! (Small plates, small baggies, etc.)

What about being more mindful while eating?

Yes, I like this idea and I think you should try to be more aware of how you feel when you are eating. Hungry or full. There are even little scales you can chart for this to help you learn to eat until you are satisfied not full. You don't need to only count on this mindfulness because sometimes our minds wander, or if you are like me my mind wanders ALL the time. Use environment manipulation to your advantage.

This can sound like a weak strategy, environment manipulation, but it can be massive! Imagine each little tweak may help you eat 10% less or 7% less or 20% less. As you add all those together you have some significant numbers. Now this tactic does not provide huge and fast weight loss because you would absolutely notice that missing food but if a couple tweaks cause you to lose 1 pound per month 12 months later being 12 pounds lighter without a big hairy fight doesn't sound too bad. These strategies are a big reason why weight maintenance is so easy for me.

To get more of your creative environment design juices flowing I will again recommend reading the Books "mindless eating" and "slim by design." Brian Wansink is hilarious and the experiments they do are very entertaining. They are available in audio form as well so you can listen while you burn calories. Good luck and skinny up your house!

<u>18</u>
Stress Effects

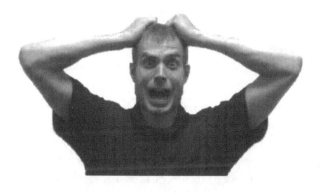

Stress is probably one of the biggest obstacles of not just weight loss but living a happy and healthy life in all categories. When I mention having less stress I'm not talking about living a life without challenges and obstacles. There is positive stress. It even has a name, eustress. Eustress is not defined by the stressor but how you perceive the stressor. This means when losing a job, one person jumps on the challenge and finds a better one while the other lands on the couch face first into a bag of chips! It's the same stressor but different perceptions. One person sees it as an opportunity and the other thinks it's the end of the world. Negative stress is called distress and involves the person being unable to cope with the stressor which causes them to act crazy (my definition). Crazy of course is not the right word but they are certainly no longer the boss of their emotions.

This was the most helpful list that explained stress to me. I'll share it with you. I saw this in a lecture at a conference

Fitness in Real Life

by Dr. Len Kravitz from University of New Mexico. Thanks a bunch Len!

Our Bodies Reaction to Stress:
When you feel challenged -> Release Norepinephrine (fight hormone)
When you feel loss of control -> Release Epinephrine (flight/anxiety hormone)
When you feel defeated -> Release Cortisol (chronic cortisol = belly fat and illness)

What this means to me is…if I feel stressed and capable I will fight. If I keep fighting but I'm clearly losing and after doubling or tripling my effort I'm still losing I will want to run! If I cannot run and the stress keeps bearing down on me I will collapse. If life makes me feel defeated and trapped too much of the time I will feel horrible and my waist might grow and arteries might clog.

To be honest I'm dealing with this as I write this book! I've been trying to bring some of these concepts to a book for 10 years now. Sometimes the concept has gotten too big so instead of finishing I've run away for a while. How will I make it this time? The same way I make it through a 5k. The day before I'm super positive and ready to crush it. As the pressure builds I lose confidence, until on the starting line I tell myself I just want to survive. Then I just take it one step at a time and ask am I doing my best right now? How about now? Until finally it's done. I've broken the book into smaller lessons and battled each "step" at a time. I unknowingly followed the Yerkes-Dodson Curve which explains peak performance and stress.

Yerkes-Dodson Curve

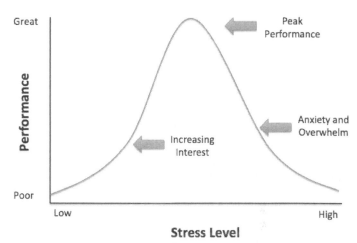

When stress is too low performance is poor. It's not important enough to care or try. When stress is off the charts performance suffers because of anxiety (flight hormone!). What we need is enough stress that it creates great performance but not so much that we buckle under the pressure. My 5k starting line thoughts of "just do your best", lower the stress level down from getting a PR (personal record). In this stressed but not over stressed spot I can then perform my best.

How you "FEEL" matters!!!

The same stress can cause positive action or paralyzing inaction depending on how you FEEL about it. If you feel challenged but positive hello peak performance but if you feel anxious, out of control, or defeated you will not perform well. Does this means stress is complicated? You betcha! You already knew that. We need to coach ourselves like we would coach our kids. We need to add excitement into an activity that is important but they are bored with and we need to let them know it's not the end of the world if they fail at something they are feeling a lot of pressure on. (My wife coaches me like this all the time!)

Who cares about stress, why not just suck it up and soldier on?

Weight gain and belly fat are just a couple reasons why you wouldn't want to just soldier on through chronic stress. Our physiology doesn't know why we are under chronic stress, only our brain knows that. Our body reacts to chronic stress the same way just more intensely depending now how intense our FEELINGS are about it.

This means for some of us:

- Being in a war zone = same as High debt load
- Attacked by a bear = same as Argument with spouse
- Living on top of active volcano = same as Juggling too many responsibilities
- Trapped under a rock = same as Trapped by Life

Our internal reaction is survival based. If we were in any of the first situations survival makes sense but the second situations in a non-emotional place we know we will survive. When stress is cronic cortisol, our stress hormone, causes us to release fat into our blood (high cholesterol anyone?) Then relocate fat into abdomen (protect organs from injury, more padding). Build new fat cells or fill existing cells by increasing appetite. One hormone, Grehlin that is responsible for appetite skyrockets the higher it goes the hungrier you get (think growling Grehlin!) Another hormone drops called Leptin. Decreased Leptin tells the body you aren't fat enough so it should gain more. So your increased hunger helps you gain more weight.

These are just some of the effects of stress I could go on but let's go to the next section and figure out how to deal with it.

19

Stress Management and Boundaries

When you are stressed, angry, or hurt it is a signal that something isn't quite right. I like the term boundary, from the book "Boundaries" by Henry Cloud to describe this. Basically, a boundary was violated and that is why you feel that way. I can't think of any reason you could feel that way without a boundary violation.

<u>Examples of Boundary Violations:</u>
Someone punches you in the face – physical boundary (personal space) & emotional boundary of feeling safe.
Someone shows up late to dinner – violated a time boundary & an emotional "I respect your time" boundary.
You get fired from your job – The boundary of YOUR JOB got violated. You saw it as yours and it got taken.
You don't like taking calls from Aunt Marge because she keeps going on and on – Your personal time is violated even if you never communicated a need to get off the phone because you feel guilty telling her that since she lives all alone. (You still feel annoyed.)
You say yes when you mean no – you say yes again to coaching the soccer team even though you don't have time and your family needs to see you more.

Types of Boundaries:

Clear Boundaries – Are like a house with a nice wooded fence around the yard. Everyone can see the boundary and they know it's there. When they go through the gate they know they are on your property. If you invite someone in you don't get upset that they are there. If someone barges in and starts cooking on your grill you might feel violated.

Unstated Boundaries – These are common and VERY common to stumble through in the first year of marriage. These are boundaries that you have but you haven't told anyone. You might let someone violate them for years getting more and more annoyed until you freak out! Like when Aunt Marge calls and you listen to her rant for over an hour AGAIN! You haven't told her but the boundary is still very real to you.

Cultural Boundaries – Whether family culture or national culture there are things that we grow up with that we assume every other person or family operates that way. Like kissing family members good-bye on lips. I grew up in a hug family but some people grew up in a kiss family. A kiss to anyone but Sarah (my wife) and my daughter Anna feels like a violation of my personal space though it may be perfectly comfortable with someone else.

Excessive Boundaries – This is a boundary that actually covers someone else's legitimate boundary. If I decided that my neighbor's lawn needs to be cut lower and I go over and cut it I'm on their property uninvited messing around with stuff. They might not care but they also might and they have every right to tell me to bug off! This can be a parent who shields a child from all challenges and difficulty, taking on their child's personal challenges that they need to solve.

Two Types of People Who Are Really Bad at Boundaries: (though all of us have played these roles occasionally)

Boundary Doormats – These people let others walk all over them without even mentioning they don't like it. This makes other people violaters even though they didn't know there was a boundary. These people are often very beaten down but also very frustrated (stressed). They sometimes snap!

Boundary Busters – These people are usually narcissists or codependents. They have a tough time thinking of other people and so blast through even well stated boundaries. They completely obliterate the Boundary Doormats. The codependents do this thinking they are helping the narcissists do this because it suits their own needs.

Basically the problem comes from someone stepping into an area physically, verbally, emotionally, etc. that someone else feels is theirs and the intrusion is not appreciated. So with this terminology you can hopefully see the stress a little differently. When you feel those negative emotions is there an excessive boundary you have placed where you shouldn't? Have you not stated your boundaries clear enough so people know where they are? Is there someone you need to be more firm with and give consequences for boundary violations?

Boundary Busting Examples Specific to Weight Loss:

- Your spouse starts making or bringing home desserts just as you start your weight loss program. Sometimes this is on purpose and sometimes it is subconscious. Either way it often means your improvement makes them feel less important.

- You get harassed at the family picnic because you brought some of your own food so you could stick to your healthy eating pattern. Usually it is their insecurity coming out.

- Your spouse keeps asking or taking you to dinner out.

Practical Ideas for Working With Stress From Boundaries:

- Read the book "Boundaries" by Henry Cloud – WAY MORE INFO!

- Let go and let God – Easier said than done. Some things are too big for us to carry. This most likely needs to be told to the codependent as they tend to take on the problems of the world. Let go of taking responsibility for everyone around you and let God handle it. I'm often in need of this reminder.

- Remember that a YES is really a NO to something else – A yes to being soccer coach is a no to more time with your family. Make sure it fits your priorities.

- "No, is a complete sentence" – Chris Charleton – Chris is actually the counselor we have really connected well with. He told me this because I always feel I need some super amazing reason in order to say no to someone. www.interactcounseling.com

- Purposefully Decrease Expectations – Sometimes you need to do this because out of this world expectations get you hurt a lot. If you expect everyone you know to call you on your birthday…ouch…you will have a sad day! You don't want to lower your expectations so much that you are thankful when someone kicks you, but sometimes you need to drop them a little.

- Journal when you feel emotions rise up – Try to find what feelings and boundaries might be involved. Daily journaling is an important step to emotional health.

- Sit down talks with boundary violators – If you are really wounded in this way it would be wise to see a counselor first. They may not have even been aware of how you felt about things. Speak the truth with love. Find a healthy vent for frustrations first.

- Build your life around your priorities – Drop more things off your schedule. Put more things you LOVE in there. Stress will decrease.

If stress is a big, often occurring struggle for you this could be the most important thing to work on in your fitness journey. It could be more powerful than a personal trainer and a perfect meal plan. Remember your body will get leaner from the brain down.

20
Sleep till you're skinny?

We all like sleep...well at least I assume we do. I haven't had too many conversations otherwise! If you don't love sleep let me give you some ideas why you should!

Why Sleep?
- **Immune System** – Enough sleep can make immune system 3x stronger compared to not enough sleep.
- **Weight Gain** - Lack of sleep causes Leptin hormone decrease and Grehlin hormone increase. We get more hungry! If our body isn't well rested it has to run on the energy of stimulants like sugar and caffeine to get through the day. This will not make you skinny I can guarantee that!
- **Memory** - When we sleep our brain does the "filing of memories". It is an organizational time for the brain. Better filing = better retrieval.
- **Clearer Thinking** - We are less foggy and spacey when we get enough sleep.
- **Better Mood** - Avoid the crankiness that comes from lack of sleep. Have you ever gotten into an argument

when you and your spouse are tired? Also sleep deceases psychological disorders like depression and paranoia. That's something you wouldn't mind having less of.

- **Decease Accidents** - 1 in 5 traffic accidents are related to lack of sleep. What about stubbing your toes? I bet there is a decrease in that too.
- **Less Pain** - or at least decreased pain sensitivity. Speaking of stubbing your toes…when you are tired you are significantly more likely to fall down crying and helpless after stubbing your toes! (Not specifically stated in researched but I think you've been there.) You are also less likely to get mad at inanimate objects.
- **Better Sex Life** - Certainly our mood is elevated. What would happen to marriage bedrooms around the world if spouses were no longer "too tired?" CRAZINESS!!!
- **Sickness** - Increased risk of serious medical issue if you are lacking sleep - ALL CATEGORIES!

One of those reasons is valuable enough to consider getting more sleep but ALL of them together mean we had better figure this out!

How Much Sleep?

From my personal research I've noticed a convergence of mental health benefits and physical health benefits that seem to agree on more than 6 1/2 hours and less than 8 1/2 hours so the ideal of **7 1/2 seems to be fair**. That also takes into account research on 90-minute sleep cycles.

Two biggest factors in sleep are time available and sleep quality. I see both of these issues happening to my clients fairly evenly. I can't tell you one is a bigger issue than the other. As far as time available we are always trying to fit more into each day and sleeping feels like a waste of time. Watch out for this trap. It's more of that short-term gain traded in for long-term pain. I've learned this one often. I'll try to fit more work into the late evening and I spend 3 hours doing something I could spend 45 minutes on if I were rested. There are other things you can probably cut that will have a bigger effect on time available than sleep. Hopefully the list above is reason enough to start allowing more time for sleep. What if you have 8 or 9 hours set aside for sleep but you aren't sleeping during that time? What if you are just lying there getting agitated?

How to improve Sleep Quality:

- **No caffeine** – Caffeine elevates stress hormones and blocks sleep (and sleep quality). Try for a minimum goal of no caffeine after noon. Ideally none of course. Caffeine's half-life in the body is 6 hours. The average cup of coffee is at least 100mg of caffeine. This means if you drink 4 cups of coffee at 6 am you will still have a cup of coffee worth of caffeine in your system at 6 pm. And ½ a cup of coffee worth of Caffeine in your body at mid-night!

- **Exercise** - Endorphins and a tired body lead to good sleep. Just don't exercise right before bed.

- **No big meal before bed** – Could create indigestion, heartburn, and excess energy. Eating less before bed means a less active stomach and fewer interruptions as well as not giving you too much energy when you are trying to shut down. (side note: check for food sensitivities)

- **Consistent time** - Keeping bedtime and wake time consistent is very important for sleep quality. It takes several days to recover sleep from the 1-2+ hour shift that occurs on the weekend. Don't give yourself jet lag every weekend!

- **Drink water earlier in the day** - Don't drink too much water before bed. Because....well you know! You might be interrupted to pee!

- **Treat your injury** - Pain from injuries are a big obstacle. Seek treatment for issues you are having. Before bed is the time of day I think painkillers can be most helpful. Don't over do it during the day and pay for it all night. Avoid painkillers for workouts so you don't over do it!

- **SUPER DARK, NICE AND COOL, Quiet or white noise** - These are important factors in ideal sleeping. A hot summer night is not good for sleep.

- **Ease into sleep** - Create a bedtime routine that includes no phone, TV, or bright light before bed (the light stimulates the brain making it get into the rhythm of day light), Make sure bathroom is dimly lit. Maybe set a go to bed alarm so you can get there on time! Give yourself time in this quiet dim environment.

- **Plan, Organize, and Prioritize to control stress** - This is probably the biggest obstacle of sleep (as well as many other issues of health and happiness).

  - Learn how decrease stress (boundaries to decrease exposure to stress)

  - Learn to vent - (exercise, safe friend, walk in woods for perspective, etc)

  - Learn to process stress - (counseling, God, helpful books)

- **Get Wise counsel** - consider a Sleep study – You can do a cheap version by tracking sleep with your exercise tracking device (most track sleep too, or at least try to). If sleep doesn't come and you lay in bed a lot I recommend a sleep study to make sure you don't have something else physiological going on, once that's ruled out then counseling may be the next option. Life does not have to be that hard. (It's hard but it doesn't need to be THAT hard ALL the time!)

- **If you do find yourself awake…**the more you get upset about it the less you'll sleep. Use that time to practice meditation or prayer. Even if you don't sleep you will "rest" and that will be helpful. Many times a calm focus on prayer or meditation will send you slowly back to sleep.

If you don't get enough sleep you have a high probability of becoming a fat crazy person! Your hunger will skyrocket and your happiness with plummet. Studies can even link poor sleep with schizophrenia, depression, and bipolar disorder. Money, stuff, busyness, etc. do not matter in the face of physical health and mental sanity. Being average in money and stuff but above average in health and happiness is a far greater goal to shoot for. Do whatever it takes to get better at sleep. Your current and long-term health and happiness rest on your pillow.

21
Create a Craving

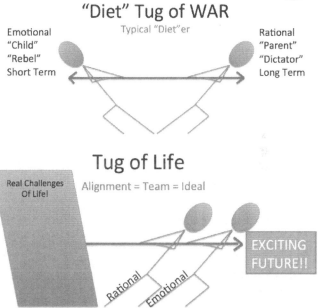

To beat a craving sometimes you need to create a craving. One of my favorite thought leaders is Dave Ramsey. He is a financial guru who's biblically based common sense principles have helped my wife and I live with very little financial stress and I love him for it. He has a radio talk show with about 6 million listeners and several books. When talking finances couples often call into his show and they are not on the same page when it comes to finances. They are actually pulling in opposite directions. Often one is the "saver" and one is the "spender". It turns out we all have both of these personalities inside us! (Well at least these two maybe more! :o)

Fitness in Real Life

The top picture is the Diet Tug of War. You can see the tension between these two sides. The emotional side which can be called our child like personality, a rebel, a spender and more interested in fun in the moment. And our rational side which can be called the parent, dictator, saver, and long-term thinker. They are of different strengths in different people. You can see how both are important. Without the "childlike" side life wouldn't be much fun. It would be safe and clean but not fun. And without the "parentlike" side bills won't get paid and you might get thrown out on the street. The problem happens when these sides are working against each other instead of with each other like in the bottom picture. Together they are an awesome team pulling against the very real challenges of life toward an exciting future and fun present.

Take a guess at which one would call into a financial radio show to get advice?

The "parent/rational" partner right? Yep, by far that is the spouse who calls because that's the side thinking more future. That's also the side that's frustrated when finances are out of control and the couple is in debt up to their eye balls. They call in and often complain how their spouse won't get on the same page about living below their means and paying off their out of control debt. Typically their approach to their fun loving spouse is, "We have to get this under control so for the next 3 years we are going to stop going out to eat, sell the nice car and buy a junker, sell all our stuff, live in a dump, and work 2-3 jobs each to get out of debt." Guess how excited the childlike partner gets? NOT EXCITED AT ALL!!! That's sounds horrible so they sink in their heals and hope the partner gives up on the craziness soon!

21 – Create a Craving

On a diet this looks like, "starting today there is a new sheriff in town. There will be no more eating things that are tasty, you will give up all your favorite foods, no eating out, no eating after 7 pm, and all you can eat is broccoli, grilled chicken, and water."

Our other personality freaks out! "This sounds horrible I hope this craziness ends soon!" And the fight is on. This is a similar description as the emotional eating section and is so important it needs to be viewed from both of these angles.

The solution?

Create a Craving

You need to paint an exciting picture of the future first then and only then reveal the simple steps to get there. My favorite activities for this is a goal body activity and vision board. Both sound really weird but our emotions can be weird sometimes. Appealing rationally to the emotional side doesn't work. Facts and figures don't fire up the engine. And our emotional engine is FAR more powerful than our rational engine.

These two activities can go together as the goal body can be part of the vision board. The goal body activity is basically pasting your head on your goal physical self. It can be a picture from the past (as long as it's not high school) or someone else's body that inspires you. The key is that it inspires you. It gets you fired up. If you feel hopeless when you look at it you need to redo it. On this vision board you can link up all the positives having this healthy body will bring to your life. Family fun, success at work, more intimacy with spouse, etc. This is a very personal activity but very powerful. When you see the benefits of this healthy body work you have EMOTIONAL energy to tackle the challenges.

The choice of saying no to a cookie is no longer a choice to go without and suffer on a "diet" but a choice to have more energy, passion, and fun! The positive desire of the future can sometimes out weigh the yummy of the moment. It won't always. Sometimes you will have the cookie but you'll notice you will be more selective in your treats because it better be REALLY good to win over the long term health and fun. Remember as you go through this process that you need fun in your life too. Don't get too strict or this will back fire. Read the want to vs have to and emotional eating sections to get a better understanding of these concepts.

If you can get your rational and emotional side working together there is nothing you won't be able to do!

Example of a vision board:
Keeping myself strong and healthy as I double my age means:

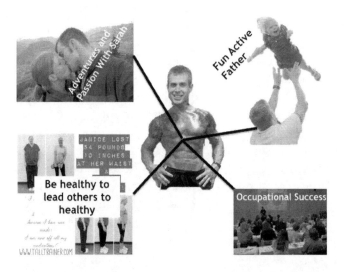

22

How to Get Rich and Lose Weight

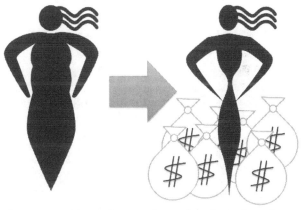

Are there two things that are hyped and marketed as much as "get rich quick" and "lose weight quick?" Financial insecurity and body insecurity are massive wounds many of us carry. When someone says they can take the pain away instantly we want to believe them even though we know it's a trick. Why does it always end up being a trick?

Consider the source

The best place to get financial advice is from someone who's got the money you wish you had. The best place for weight loss advice is from someone who has done it and kept it off. Not a celebrity who endorses a new weight loss trick every couple years because they gained all their weight back from the last time. We also know better than to take financial advice from the lotto winners. They don't have a repeatable or long-term successful plan. Celebrities go broke all the time in-spite of millions of dollars and people gain back their weight even after surgeries! Another important point is don't take lessons from only one person who is successful. You need to know what works every time consistently. The best source of information on getting rich is the book called "The Millionaire Next Door" by Thomas J. Stanley and William D. Danko. It turns out most millionaires aren't who you think they are. Celebrities and sports only make up 1% of millionaires. Who are these people? What do they do? How can I be like them? All that and more is answered in the book. What about the best source for long-term weight loss advice? Currently one of the best sources is the national weight control registry (www.nwcr.ws). Feedback from thousands of people who have lost weight and kept it off. You will find what I say here will not conflict with the information you find there.

My financial coach told me...

Dave Ramsey is my top financial coach and he is for about 6-7 million other people as well. His book "The Total Money Makeover" is a must read for every person on the planet. He has 7 steps to financial peace and prosperity. They are all very basic. It turns out that's the truth of getting rich. It's also the truth about losing weight and being healthy. Simple but not easy.

There is one thing that people who are successful with money and people who are successful with their body weight do (especially if they have struggled in the past). This is actually the engine that makes Dave's advice work. Without it people are lost, confused, stressed, and perpetually stuck.

KEEP A WRITTEN BUDGET

22 – How to Get Rich and Lose Weight

For your finances you need to designate where your money is going to go for the month so you aren't asking yourself at the end of the month where it went. The same goes for food/calories. You need to plan your eating so you get to the end of the day without breaking your budget!

Is this fun to do? Not for most people. Is it rewarding to do? Absolutely! Sarah and I paid off $98,000 in debt in the first 3.5 years of marriage. Yes, we sometimes ate beans and rice and we lived in a trailer for some of that time. Dave says, "live like no one else so later you can live and give like no one else." With $1,200 fewer bills each month it's like getting a raise. And financial stress drops away! What about weight loss? This food journal thing isn't easy. But it's so worth it. Imagine being at your goal weight without having any more weight to lose. You look great. You feel healthy. You have energy and smiles that brighten the world around you. This is a proven way to get rich and lose weight EVERYTIME! In weight loss studies people who keep a food journal lose twice as much weight as those who don't! Oh man I want that!

If you've been in DEBT this goes double for you...

We all know the people who don't keep a record of their money but are doing just fine. We also know people who don't keep track of their food and they do just fine as well. These people aren't like you. They've never struggled. They don't have as many habits to change. If you've been overweight or in debt you know that you don't feel like you have a handle on this area. You NEED a budget to learn about money and/or about calories so you can get a handle on this.

While I recommend a monthly financial budget for every month you plan to be alive, I think you can take breaks from your food journaling. This isn't a life sentence. Many people can get to their goal weight and maintain for a few months and slowly let up on the journal and maintain for a while. When the bumps of life come in and you notice your pants getting tighter or the scale getting heavier it might be time to get back to it.

How to food journal

Keeping track of Calories is the bare minimum. To do this you need to weigh and measure your food and keep a record on paper or better yet use food journaling software (because it's easier). We use one with our clients that calculates vitamins and minerals as well as macronutrients so you get to learn not just how to lose weight but how to eat healthfully.

1. Buy digital food scale
2. Pour or place food on scale to measure in grams
3. Compare to package label and write calories down or enter into software
4. Use this information to follow other guidelines in this book = success

If you want to do this right, I want to help. I can give you a free 1-week trial of our food journaling software so you can see how this can work and get a big boost. Contact us at www.talltrainer.com/31lessonsbook

23

Nerd Out With Numbers

Here are some helpful numbers that can assist you in understanding the body, weight loss, and health.

Type of Macronutrient	Calories/Gram	Calories in 100g
Carbohydrate	4	400 Calories
Protein	4	400 Calories
Fat	9	900 Calories
Alcohol	7	700 Calories

Mistakes people make once they know these numbers.

1.) They think 100g of chicken has 100g of protein. Not so; there is water, minerals, even some carbohydrate and fat in the chicken too. A good food journal software can help you track these Macronutrients in your food.

2.) They see 9 Calories/gram of Fat and decide not to eat any of that. BIG mistake because out body needs fat and it helps us to be more full. You do need to watch out! I've known plenty of people that have killed their Calories for the day with a "couple handfuls of almonds."

3.) They think Carbohydrates only come in breads. Carbohydrates are in fruits and vegetables too and are very important for health. I don't mind people being low on "bread type" carbs but not low carbs by skipping veggies.

4.) This isn't necessarily a mistake but isn't it shocking that alcohol is like liquid butter as far as Calorie content? It's also digested in the liver like a lot of our fats.

5.) Macronutrients like Protein, Carbohydrates, and Fat are not the only thing our bodies need. Don't forget about vitamins and minerals. This is why our food journaling software is so useful it helps us see those levels too.

Calories in a pound of Fat: 3,500 Calories
Calories burned in walking or running a mile: About 100 Calories

These are helpful numbers to know because:

- When you eat a little more on the weekend and you are up 4 pounds you know that you didn't eat 14,000 extra calories above your metabolism. There is likely some fluid retention that will stay until that food has worked it's way out.

- When you eat a little less for a couple days you probably didn't eat 3,500 less so you may not lose a pound until you keep it up longer.

- When you go for a 5 mile run or walk and you aren't down a pound or two you can know that the 5 miles was only $1/7^{th}$ of a pound as far as Calories burned. (Don't eat the 700 Calories of ice cream to celebrate!)

- If you want to lose 20 pounds that is 70,000 Calories you need to burn and not eat. At an ambitious 1,000 Calories per day (burn 2,500 eat 1,500) it will take you 70 days to get those 20 pounds off. (This is why we need a lifestyle change not just a "diet". It's hard to lose weight!)

- Fun Fact: Since there are 3,500 Calories in a Pound and 365 Days a year you can easily guestimate long-term effects of consistent Calories lost. If you are eating 100 Calories per day less than your Calories burned consistently for a year you can move the decimal point over to get the estimate. 100.0 Cals/Day = 10 pounds/year (roughly). Long math: 100 Cals X 365 = 36,500 Calories ÷ 3,500 Cals/pound = 10.4 pounds over the year! 500 Calories per day different? = 50 pounds over the year!

Percent of Calories used in Digestion:

500 Calories of	% burned in digestion	Calories burned in digestion	Calories available for body
Protein	20-30%	150	350
Carbohydrate	5-18%	Veg = 90	410
		Sweets = 25	475
Fat	0-3%	15	485

This information is must useful to see the benefits of a diet high in protein and vegetables. Veggies use closer to 18% of Calories in digestion compared to breads and sweets, which are closer to 5%. You burn more calories in digestion so you store less fat!

Basic Macronutrient Targets:

Macronutrient	Percent of Calories	Calorie Range (for 2,000 Cals)	Grams (for 2000 Cals)
Carbohydrate	45-65%	900-1,300 Cals	225-325 g
Protein	10-35%	200-700 Cals	50-175 g

Fat	20-35%	400-700 Cals	44-78 g

Using this info let's see what two different days could cost for digestion Calories: (using 2,000 Calorie Diets)

Option 1:
65% Calories from Sweets = 1,300 Calories = 65 Calories in digestion
10% Calories from Protein = 200 Calories = 60 Calories in digestion
25% Calories from Fat = 500 Calories = 10 Calories in digestion
Total Calories Used in Digestion = **135 Calories**

Option 2:
45% Calories from Veggies = 900 Calories = 162 Calories in digestion
35% Calories from Protein = 700 Calories = 210 Calories in digestion
20% Calories from Fat = 400 Calories = 8 Calories in digestion
Total Calories Used in Digestion = **380 Calories**

That's a 245 Calorie Difference!!!
This could mean 24.5 pounds lost if done daily for a year! You don't have to be this extreme either. It's still over 12 pounds lost if you are only halfway there!

Jeremy's Rule of Thumb:
This always gave me a rough idea if I was on track and a way to look at what people were eating and see if they were on track.

Protein grams are ½ of Carbohydrate grams
Fat grams are ½ of Protein grams

23 – Nerd Out With Numbers

If Carbs are 240g then protein could be near 120g and Fat near 60g

This is 1980 Calories (basically 2000) and Percentages are:

> Carbs = 48%
>
> Protein = 24%
>
> Fat = 27%

There will be some individual differences but this gives you a quick way to see if your day is on track or if a meal is roughly balanced.

Ok, you can put your calculator and pocket protector away now we are done with the numbers.

24

I overate…Why is my weight down?

If this happens to you don't assume you found the new ice cream and pasta diet that will help you lose gobs of weight (if only it were true). This is however a very important concept for us to understand if we seek long term success in weight loss and maintenance.

Carbohydrate Cycling for Sustained Weight Loss

If you are on a "diet" for a week you will probably lose weight. If you are on it for 3 weeks you will probably lose weight. At some point you will be still on a "diet" and your weight will get stuck. There are a dozen reasons for this but right now I just want you to learn about one that could be a factor.

We will have answers to these troubling problems:
• I overate…why is my weight down?
• I'm not losing weight anymore and I'm still eating 1200 Calories per day!
• My skinny friend can eat whatever they want and not get FAT!

You Need to Meet Leptin…

Leptin is a hormone in our body that tells our body that we have plenty of fat so it's ok if we lose some. If you are overweight you probably have a high leptin level. This means the first few pounds will be easier to lose than the last few pounds. The only other way I know of currently to have a high leptin level is to eat as if you ate like this everyday you would be overweight. So you eat a few more calories and maybe a special treat. Now if we eat this way everyday guess what?…(no rocket science needed)…We will be overweight! This doesn't seem like a good solution to any of these problems.

Here's how it works. Imagine that I have been on my weight loss plan strict and strong for a couple weeks. I lost some weight and now I'm stuck. This happens sooner for those closer to their goal weight (less body fat to keep leptin up). If you are obese you can sometimes make it through several months of weight loss before this becomes an issue. Anyway you have not "cheated" or let your guard down but still your weight loss slows and may even stop. First wait a minimum 1 week at this level (prefer 2 weeks). If it's still stuck then this high eating day might boost your leptin levels to create weight loss again! **IMPORTANT: ONE DAY ONLY!!!**

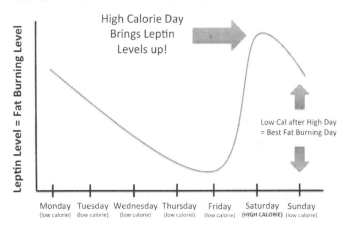

The day after a high calorie and high carb day is your peak fat loss day. Get back on plan ASAP! Be strong because you may notice extra hunger that day. Fight the cravings with protein and vegetables early and often.

So this answers the problem "I'm not losing weight anymore..." and "I overate...why is my weight down?" Sometimes this happens by accident. Let's say we've been really strong on our "diet" and we have been eating low carb and low calories for weeks now. But, we have a weak moment and eat several slices of pizza. As we are beating ourselves up the next day we step on the scale and we lost!! We think perhaps we have discovered a Pizza Diet or Ice Cream diet. This is not the case you just gave yourself an accidental high day and boosted your leptin levels so your body said, "ok you can go away" to some more body fat!

How we react determines success or failure. If we have a high day (or weak moment if unplanned) and we give up on our eating plan because we blew it and take on a weekend long anything goes attitude then we won't lose weight. However, if we see it for what it is and get back on plan we can see continued success.

What about the friend who can eat anything they want?

Well you might see them on their "high days". Oftentimes a skinny friend may not have to be as conscious of their weight because they are more intuitive with their bodies. When they are more hungry it's because they are actually hungry not because of emotions or stress. So some days they are too busy to eat that much and other days they eat a lot more. The net effect is a high leptin level occasionally and fat loss on the low calorie days. They might eat more than you when you are together but I'll bet if we had a private investigator follow them around and you around they would find the skinny friend averaging fewer calories and you hitting a much higher level more often.

Important Tips if you want to try this out:
- Make sure you know for sure you've been at a low calorie level. If you're not at a low level eating more for a day will just make you gain weight. (I suppose you'll know if it's helpful or not if you find yourself gaining). Keep a food journal and measure your food to be sure.
- After a high day sometimes you are down the next day other times it might take 3 days for it to show up. Don't assume it's a flop until you wait a week and see if your weight is down from the week previous. (your weight might go up for a day or two before it goes down)
- For a beginner at this I recommend 1 day per week. There are more tricks but starting with one day a week should help you break through enough.
- I usually tell people to eat 500-1000 Calories more than your low days.
- Aim for more carbohydrates specifically
- Protein can be lower that day too
- The day after start with a good breakfast with protein and veggies. Eat every three hours or so to avoid getting hungry on this high metabolism day. If you aren't careful you'll get hungry and have two high days in a row and that's not going to help you lose weight.
- Eating low bread type (starchy) carbohydrates through the week can help make the effect more pronounced
- Since this is getting on the outside edge of my training - Read up on this yourself...I didn't invent Leptin or Carbohydrate Cycling. I'm just telling you what I've seen work with my clients.
- This may not be a good idea for you personally. Meeting one on one with a trainer or diet professional is a GREAT IDEA!

<u>25</u>

On the Other Side of No There is Joy

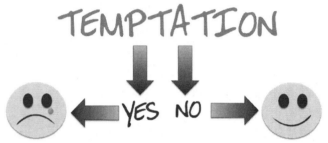

Our temptations whether they are food, sex, alcohol, gambling, work, and other good things used incorrectly all lie to us. They tell us do _____ because it will make you happy. It's exciting. Tasty. Fulfilling. And for a few brief moments they are. We indulge in our temptation and get our fill/fix. Then what?

If you are like me then a feeling of regret takes the place of the all too brief enjoyment. I've had this happen to me simply watching television. It promised me a break from my stressed and busy mind. "I'll just watch a little," is what I tell myself. "I've worked hard I DESERVE a mental break." Hours later when I finally muster the willpower to shut it off, what am I left with? All the stressors I had before I watched TV AND now I have less time so I am even more stressed.

If food is a temptation for you think back to your last emotional eating encounter. The food promised to be yummy and take the stress or sadness away. When you

118

finished eating and came back out of your eating bliss, did you have less stress or perhaps more because your weight is one of your stressors?

"Eat what makes you happy!"

I overheard a couple ladies at a restaurant. (I try not to eavesdrop but the conversation was loud and the topic felt like work.) That was the advice being dolled out. I agree and disagree. The statement is too vague. Eat what makes you happy right now? Eat what makes you happy when you try on clothes? Eat what makes you happy at the doctor's office?

I want you happy.

Not for minutes or hours and then you feel worse. I want you happy for a lifetime. There is a word you use to help bring in that long-term happiness. We don't say it enough. It can bring unspeakable joy into your life.

That word is "NO!"

"On the other side of No there is JOY!"
– Pastor Bill Bambach (Life Spring Community Church, Canandaigua, NY, www.lifespringcc.com)

When we say no to a temptation (food or other) we might feel a little sad at first that we missed a big time high. After the quick sadness there is a feeling of control, power, and a little pride in yourself. One of my favorite moments happens often at the scale when we weigh someone in before a workout. Someone begins describing this amazing dessert that everyone around them was eating. They look at me like they just hit a home run to win the World Series and say, "And I didn't have any!" They were not sad. They had just lost weight, gotten healthier, AND boosted their confidence into the stratosphere (that's like WAY up there). The twinkle in their eye, smile on their face, and spring in their step most definitely said "On the other side of No there is JOY!"

There is a time and a place for an outright NO! A word of caution for some of us, we can start to feel bullied if it feels like we are saying NO against our will (see emotional eating section). This is why most diets end in a binge and people gain back most of the weight they lost. It's not "NO." It's just not today. This is similar to the approach at Alcoholics Anonymous as the big goal is to be sober today not for the next year. Saying never ever ever for the rest of my life I will not have a cookie takes too much willpower. Saying not today is a little easier. This strategy coupled with the carbohydrate cycling we already learned about could have us say no for a few days then say yes on our high day. However, if you notice that when you say yes you end up eating 2 dozen cookies you are an excellent candidate for more reading, journaling, a support group, and counseling. You can get through it but pretending it can be solved by the next "diet" is a recipe for many more years of struggle.

We do need to be able say no sometimes. There are just too many opportunities for extra Calories that we can come across in one day. It is so important that we don't buy into the lies of the temptation. I'll leave you with 3 questions from Zig Ziglar's book "Courtship After Marriage: Romance That Lasts a Lifetime." He said to **try asking yourself these 3 questions before you indulge in any pleasure.**

1. Can I repeat this pleasure indefinitely and be happy?
2. Would I be willing for the person I love the most to see me doing this?

25 – On the Other Side of No There is Joy

    3.   Will this pleasure be at someone else's expense?

If you can answer positively to these questions then enjoy that moment of pleasure. If you can't answer positively to these questions then on the other side of that "NO" is long-term Joy.

26

Momentum

An object at rest tends to stay at rest until a force acts on it. An object in motion tends to stay in motion until a force acts on it. This momentum equation helps us understand how objects move in a frictionless environment.

$$\left(\frac{\textbf{Focused Intensity}}{\textbf{TIME}} \right) \times \textbf{GOD} = \textbf{Momentum}$$

Momentum is also a big deal for our lives and our habits (especially healthy one's!) This formula is from Dave Ramsey, from his business book and course called "Entreleadership": Focused intensity over time multiplied by God = Momentum. We've all experienced momentum in our lives. When you have a habit of exercise going and it just becomes your routine or on the other side you've been on a couch after work and you want to add exercise in but you just can't seem to get yourself going. Life feels better when you have momentum on your side.

Two ways to get momentum started - Impact vs. Progression

I can't tell you which one of these is better for you but I think it's a combination of both. We run a once a year team weight loss contest called Thinner to Winner that creates a 6-week momentum blaster for many people. Some people will have a life change after that 6-weeks of focused intensity and never look back. Other people will make changes that they quickly abandon once the challenge is over and gain all the weight back and then some. A final group will get so intimidated by the amount of change that they don't really participate in the challenge. This 6-week challenge is an example of an impact. Like balls on a pool table hit each other and transfer momentum suddenly. There are weight loss reality shows that use this same tactic.

Going from couch potato to signing up for a workout program can be a similar sudden boost of momentum. Some people will join our program and want a full meal plan that they can eat. We get them a plan and they only eat that. They get to every workout and have record setting results in one month. For some this new style of eating and exercise sticks long term and they never look back. I'd love to say that's what happens with most people. That is rare. The majority hit an amazing level of success then leave those habits because they are "done".

For the people who get overwhelmed at the 6-week fitness challenge and don't take action and the people who lose but then gain back a longer duration plan is needed.
Small consistent steps may be the way to go. It won't be massive change at first but consistent force over time will create momentum. This is like pushing a car from a dead stop. You push hard but only get a little motion if you keep pushing it slowly gets faster and faster until you are jogging to keep up! This only works if the force stays consistent. If you push that car for 3 sec every 5 minutes you will not build momentum. It will roll, stop, roll, stop and never get anywhere significant. For these people we work on one strategy at a time, Water, Protein, Logging Food, Vegetables, etc. Once they master one area and make a habit we can work on the next. This strategy works better for more people. Long term success is more likely using this tactic.

Fitness in Real Life

Focus your focus

Dave Ramsey's momentum theorem says "focused" intensity over time. If you try to workout everyday, drink more water, eat more protein, eat more vegetables, eat every 3-4 hours, and on and on you are in danger of being unfocused. There are too many things to work on at once! You do some of those things some of the time and make no progress. You may shift focus from career, social activities, hobbies, to focus on your physical health but you need to focus that focus. Pick a small area to REALLY focus on. Push that water car until it's rolling faster than you can run (habit) and then push the protein car. This is how I have slowly improved over time and how I will continue to do so. People think I was born with my habits and that they came easy and overnight. I had to be convinced it was something I not only needed but wanted to do and then start doing it with focused intensity.

Life has friction and other disrupting forces

Once you get the car rolling whether with an impact or steady pushing there are forces that are going to slow or stop your momentum. In physics we talk about friction. This is the force that slows the car once you stop pushing. If you've got it rolling well it takes awhile to slow it significantly but that force is always there. Our good habits do need attention from time to time. Maybe our attendance at our workout class starts to slip or we start visiting the treadmill less and less often. Sure we still do it but the momentum of that habit is beginning to slow. Without checking back into it we are in danger of dropping it completely very soon. We need to stay on guard for this. In our program we have monthly goals, measurements, and even a fitness test combined with a review time. You need to create regular review for yourself to consciously look at what is working and what isn't. This will help you catch a slip before it becomes a fall.

Life disruptions

I remember my mom's journey. My mom lost weight and got to her goal but then my grandfather (her dad) died and the grief and family drama that happened afterwards caused her to gain a large amount of that weight back. She didn't have a workout class that encouraged her at the time so she went so far off she basically had to re-start (after a couple years).

- Death or Sickness of a loved one
- Health issue / Injury
- Job Loss / Change
- Relationship turmoil – kids in trouble, divorce, etc

These and about a million other things mess up our pretty habits and daily pattern all the time. When dealing with small disruptions the key is to defend your health behaviors against these distractions. Sometimes setting up a plan for distractions that keep recurring. Like having your kid buy lunch at school instead of making their lunch because they keep forgetting it at home and you have to give up your workout time to bring it to them. (Other creative solutions possible as well).

When the big disruptions come there is certainly a time and place to postpone your workout. If you are on your way to the gym and you learn your spouse was in a car accident and is being taken to the hospital it's ok to miss a workout! If a loved one is dying you may spend extra time with them and have to eat less healthy food at not the best times. If this goes on for over a week it's ok to take a couple minutes to do something for yourself too. Like grocery shop and eat a nice salad. You may stop pushing that car (habit) for a moment and it may lose momentum. As soon as you can you need to get back to it and perhaps even increase your work in that area to get it rolling full speed again.

27

Boredom is a Huge Challenge

Boredom stops us from doing the good things we need to do to be healthy and also makes us reach for unhealthy and unproductive things to soothe the discontent. There were 3 things I identified early in my career that broke up peoples good workout routine. There are certainly more but these were the big 3, Injury, Lack of Results, and Boring Workouts. I had seen it in myself and the people I trained. Fighting these 3 workout blockers became part of the mission of Tall Trainer Fitness. Our core philosophy hinges off of Safety, Results, and Fun.

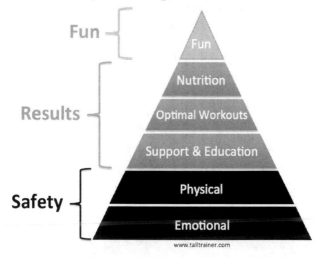

The Keys to Your Success...
Why Our Program Works.

Fun
Results
Safety

Fun
Nutrition
Optimal Workouts
Support & Education
Physical
Emotional

www.talltrainer.com

Fun is important because boring workouts don't keep people going long term. You can hit the treadmill, listen to music and stare at the wall in your basement only so many times before most of us find some reason we don't have time for that today. So how do we fight boredom at Tall Trainer?

New workouts all the time - 100's of workouts - People who have been training with us for years are still seeing new stuff. Make sure you try new exercises on a consistent basis.

Consistent strength training for 3 months then change it up. If you change too often you cannot guarantee progress. You need some repetition in your workouts to allow you to improve on some of those activities. We do the same style of resistance workout 1-2x per week then before the body and mind have a chance to get tired of it we change it.

Social - Workout with others. Laugh, joke, share life. If you aren't looking forward to sweating or burning your muscles you might look forward to seeing your exercise buddies. That will prevent boredom and keep you coming back for more.

Energy - We bring energy into our classes. If you are somewhere and the instructor looks bored themselves find a new place to workout. Find a place that gets you all sorts of fired up! We play energetic music, shout encouragement, and generally have a blast leading workouts. Find some fun and join in!

Boredom at home or boredom with life! (DANGER!)

27 – Boredom is a Huge Challenge

This is the biggest nutrition challenge for so many people. I began to identify this more and more as I noticed some people actually lose weight on vacation! My wife is usually one of those people. Every time we went on vacation she would come back lighter. I had to figure this out otherwise their weight loss program would be way too expensive (vacation all year round). I found that people on vacation eat, drink, and relax. That sounds like how most people gain weight. How are these people losing? My wife and I were able to figure out her weight loss and have investigated with others and many have found the same thing happening.

When they are on vacation they eat breakfast, lunch, and dinner out at a restaurant most of the time. They are busy, active, and entertained in between so they do not think about food. There is no fridge fully stocked or cabinets with sinful goodies hiding within reach. They lose weight because they are busy, relaxed, and constant snacking goes away. At home they might be more stressed, have these bored times, and have snacks just feet away.

I need to explain my wife a little more since she is a big reason for this discovery. My wife is 5'7" and at one time weighed in at 89 pounds as an anorexic teen. She almost died. Then she learned about bulimia and gained some weight while vomiting daily. As she worked to battle bulimia she overate her way to 189 pounds. 100 pounds in 3 years! Some of that she desperately needed. She has done a lot of work to get to the roots of these issues and structure her life to create more balance so she relies on food less. It is safe to say she is an emotional eater in a strong way (we all are at varying degrees). When we moved into our trailer after getting married she worked for over a week or two painting everything. When we moved out of the trailer a couple years later into our house she did the same thing. I learned that I need to watch out for her and actually remind her to eat in those times because she gets so busy she forgets. If you have ever starved yourself to near death over years the idea of forgetting to eat is crazy. Hunger is a scary thing to feel in your body because it nearly killed you. This is also why those starvation style diets don't work because when you are done you can't stand feeling hungry and overeat your weight back on. So, how does this woman with a huge fear of hunger forget to eat? She is so NOT bored that she doesn't need to use food to fill in the gap.

I'm convinced that God designed us for meaningful work. He did not design us to collapse on the couch after a long day of sitting at a desk staring at a light source (which I'm doing right now). Since this discovery we have found over and over again that our clients have this struggle too. If you don't have a meaningful project or work that you can't wait to get back to, the boredom causes many to look for a fun snack. These "fun" snacks add up and can easily undo your high intensity interval workout that morning or eclipse the salad you had for lunch.

How to not get bored...

House projects - When you get home get going on a fun project that allows you to see results. Ideally it uses body and mind.

Volunteer - If you have boring days volunteer in an active way. Again moving body and using mind is ideal.

Get a different job - If you spend all day bored at work you will snack more there too. Find work that inspires you.

Go play outside - Isn't that what we tell our kids?

27 – Boredom is a Huge Challenge

Plan time with friends that doesn't involve eating - A walking friend, workout friend, etc.

Get a hobby - Crafting, woodworking, making gifts for people, etc.

Pretend you are the parent of yourself and you just walked in the room saying "I'm bored", what would you suggest? Then do it! Do something weird on a regular basis. It'll bring out your silly again. Don't let your life get boring. There is truly so much cool stuff to do. Keep your workout time interesting so you keep doing it and keep the rest of the day full of fun challenging activities and you won't be looking for extra calories to fill time.

28

Want to vs. Have to

Do you HAVE to go to work?
Do you HAVE to workout?
Do you HAVE to avoid sweets?
Do you HAVE to get up early?

Well that stinks and it's a sure bet that by the end of the day you'll be exhausted doing all these things you HAVE to do. It can be easy to adopt the "poor me attitude" when faced with a busy day or a weight loss and fitness challenge. At the risk of oversimplifying something complex, all we need to do is change our mind about the activity. Changing a HAVE to into a WANT to.

You can do all the same activities, have a busy day, deal with big challenges, and end up feeling great at the end of the day.

Thoughts are PHYSICAL. They have a physical and chemical response in every cell of our bodies. Positive physical benefits for positive thoughts. Negative physical benefits for negative thoughts.

When you feel challenged -> Release Norepinephrine (fight hormone)
When you feel loss of control -> Release Epinephrine (flight/anxiety hormone)
When you feel defeated -> Release Cortisol (fat gain hormone)

These thought reactions flow throughout our entire bodies and tell our cells whether to take action or lay down and wait to die. It is how we "FEEL" about what happens to us that matters more than the actual event. Feeling challenged is awesome! It has the potential to lift us out of lethargy and get us doing something productive. If we feel overwhelmed we will not perform well and our bodies definitely bear the burden.

I WANT to workout = Challenge
I HAVE to workout = Loss of Control

I WANT to eat healthy = Challenge
I HAVE to eat healthy = Loss of Control

If you want a happier, healthier, skinnier life we need to change our thoughts. I am pretty passionate and believe in this mental shift because I needed to use it to get through a tough spot. I went through a tough time a couple years back. I had gotten a good kick to the gut by "that's just business." It was a challenge that could have closed many businesses. It hurt bad enough I wanted to crawl into a hole and die (I'm a sensitive fella). I didn't have much positivity to give to my clients. I had moments I didn't WANT TO go to work. God carried me through that phase and he kept pushing me to work not because I HAD TO but because I WANTED TO. He reminded me that it's not MY BUSINESS it's His. While I still try to take back ownership from time to time it's helpful to give some of that stress and pressure to Him.

How to find a WANT TO inside a HAVE TO:
- List all the benefits there are for the thing you want to do.
- Think through the consequences of NOT doing what you HAVE TO do.

Fitness in Real Life

- List other options instead of your HAVE TO.

<u>Let's use going to work as an example.</u>
Benefits of going to work:
- They pay you
- There might be benefits (health etc.)
- You aren't laying around watching TV being useless
- You get to interact with other people
- You ....

Consequences of not going to work:
- They stop paying you and probably end the benefits too
- You have to find something to do with 8+ hours of your day
- You won't see people as much
- Etc.

List other options instead of your HAVE TO:
It is important that you never feel stuck. Remember...there are people near the equator who live in grass and mud huts that have nothing and are probably happier than you are. If you can afford this book you could probably sell everything you have for plane tickets for you and your immediate family and settle down to a life of picking coffee beans or fishing or something else. Ok, this might not sound like something you WANT TO do but realize it's an option. When we don't have options we feel a loss of control (anxiety). So maybe you don't live in the rainforest with a loin cloth tribe, but you could downsize your house and get any old job for ½ the pay. Ok, so maybe you don't WANT TO do that either but again it's an option. You can quit your job, stop paying your bills, lose your material possessions, live on the street, or try to get government assistance. (I hope this one isn't

too appealing :o) but it is still an option. I remember the movie "Office Space" where an office worker has an existential crisis and decides not to go to work. "I don't like it so I'm just not going to go." It is a choice and a hilarious movie in my opinion.

You aren't STUCK!!!! Now that you have options you can choose. You might choose to go to work now but not because you HAVE TO but because you WANT TO. It's the choice you WANT TO make!

What got my fire for my work back again? The thought of all the people we were helping not having a place to get this kind of help. And doing the worst case scenario - realizing that if it all goes away (it could anytime) that God is good and I can probably get a better paying job in someone else's business with the level of training and work ethic I have. I reminded myself that down shifting lifestyle would not be the end of the world. Sarah and I started our marriage living in a trailer and were very happy there. I could work for minimum wage and still have a beautiful life with my wife and daughter. (That level of downshift is possible because of God inspired financial planning taught by Dave Ramsey, we have no student loans, no car payments, and no mortgage. If you are curious see www.daveramsey.com.) I woke up every morning and raced to work because I WANTED TO help people like you for as long as the doors stay open! (And I still do!)

Now go to work because you WANT TO contribute to the world.

Go exercise because you WANT TO feel strong and healthy again.

Fitness in Real Life

Eat some food that is good for you because you WANT TO be lean and energetic.

And keep reading this book because you WANT TO be inspired more.

29

Is Healthy Food Dangerous?

Is arthritis dangerous?   Is heart disease dangerous?   Is cancer dangerous?

Ok, the answer is yes. I'm only being partially dramatic here. The "healthy" food you eat could lead you down the road to some nasty issues. This is a topic I want to make sure everyone understands or has at least heard of at least once.

Food Sensitivities

I was introduced to this topic through my mother's work with a naturopathic doctor Dr. Bonnie Cronin (www.drbonniecronin.com). I had never heard of such weirdness as food sensitivities. Now we hear about dairy and gluten fairly often. My mom found out she was reacting to gluten, dairy, and nightshades! She was struggling to lose weight, had low energy, depression, and had symptoms of arthritis in her hands. If you don't understand this concept let me take a crack at it.

Food Sensitivities are like Bee Stings

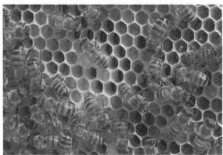

Photo: sweetbeez.org - Non-profit to help and teach about bees

Some people have no reaction and some people die. You have probably heard of people having an anaphylactic reaction to a food and a bee sting (puffing up). But those aren't the only 2 choices (zero reaction or massive reaction). There are people at every level in between. We've heard of people with food allergies or those poor kids who could die if they even touch a peanut butter molecule. That is a severe reaction, but there are less severe reactions that could still cause a problem. Our response to food can change during our life. Don't be caught off guard that you might be having a "new" food sensitivity as you age, when you are stressed, or hitting a different phase like pregnancy or menopause.

Food Sensitivities are like Sandpaper

The other way to describe this topic besides bee stings is by thinking about sand paper. The lining of our digestive system has a "skin" almost like our skin on the outside of our bodies. If you were to brush up against some sand paper once a week you would only get those white scrape marks (a scrape only in the dead skin on the surface). If you did it daily several times a day you would begin to have an open wound. If you kept at it you would be looking at infection and amputation eventually. Each individual moment is no big deal, just a little sensitive, but when you bring them all together it becomes a very big deal. If we eat a food we are sensitive to once in awhile it's no problem, our body can recover. If we eat this food daily and at high quantities our body may get behind and inflammation begins. (Stress can increase this reaction and slow healing)

We can't see inside our bodies. We can only monitor our reactions to see if something is going on. You don't want to wait for colon cancer or a heart attack until you put a stop to the inflammation.

Here are some signs you might have a food sensitivity:
- Constipation or Diarrhea (Dis-biosis)
- Low Energy
- Skin – Rashes or Breakouts
- Asthma
- Allergies
- Post Nasal Drip
- Arthritis
- Puffiness
- Weight Retention
- Head Aches
- Acid Reflux
- Anything Inflammatory

What do you do if you suspect a food sensitivity? You can go to an allergist and your sensitivity may be strong enough to be classified as an allergy and get treatment. Many of the sensitivities are just below allergy level but still have an effect.

Most common food sensitivities are:
- Dairy
- Wheat (gluten)

139

- Night Shades (Tomatoes, Potatoes, Peppers, and Eggplant)
- Sugar, Soy, Nuts, and Eggs can also be an issue.
- Basically any food that someone could be allergic to someone else could be sensitive to.

How to find out:

The gold standard would be an elimination diet where you basically eat non-night shade veggies, olive oil, organic chicken or fish, and rice or quinoa for weeks to get the body to heal and settle down. After that you bring in one new food at a time and eat it for three days to see if you react. If you don't react then you add it back into your diet and then try a different food back in for a few days. If you react you keep that food out of your diet.

This sounds too difficult for me. I have in fact never done this even though I know I have a few food issues. My strategy is that if you suspect a food is an issue you eliminate that one food from your diet for a few weeks then bring it back in large doses. If you notice you feel better with it gone you might have a sensitivity. You might not notice anything until you bring it back then with that large amount you may find yourself reacting and feeling terrible. The down side of my method is that if you have multiple food sensitivities you may not feel much better by only eliminating one food.

Personally...

I don't have much dairy because I've learned it bloats me terribly. This also means whey protein is out since it is made from dairy. I also don't have TONS of bread/gluten as I have noticed it makes me sleepy and sluggish. (I will still have both from time to time but it's less now that I know these things).

Final Thought:

Don't eliminate a food to punish yourself, but consider having it less to take care of your body. Later on you may be able to have it in small amounts. Most foods aren't worth cancer to me so I am inspired to eat them less.

30
The Key to Unhappiness
(comparing yourself to others)

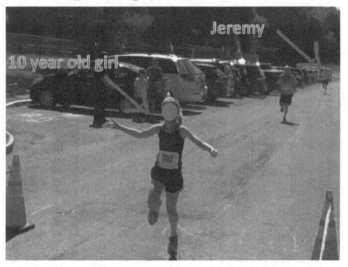

I was 33 years old on race day. I'm a personal trainer. I've been exercising for 20+ years in a serious way. I'm 6'3" and 190 pounds with 6-pack abs. My legs are LONG. My lungs can move massive amounts of air.

Why is it that a 10-year-old girl beat me in a 5k?

By all accounts I should NEVER lose to a 10-year-old girl in any feat of athletic endeavor. I'm in "my prime" as they call it. She was about 2 feet shorter than me. At most she can claim exercising for 10 years (counting learning to walk). Yet she beat me in a 5k as I ran my best time of my life up to that point, my first sub 20-minute 5k (3.1 miles)!

Ways to be unhappy in exercise:
- Believe your physical limits are very limited which then limits your achievements
- Look at others and wish you were like them
- Focus on all the things you are not able to do instead of the things you are doing

Limited Physical Limits:

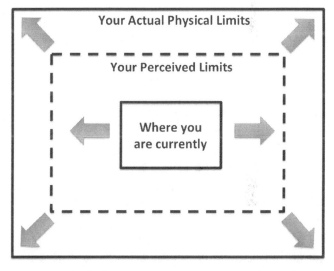

If you don't believe you have much of a chance to improve then you don't have much excitement or energy for the improvement process. The picture above is an attempt to show this concept visually. You are currently at a certain ability level. Then outside of that is a dashed line around that which is your perceived limits. If you don't have much hope or belief then your dashed line will be very close to your current state. Not much opportunity for growth. Then WAY outside of that dashed line is your actual physical limit. There is one there but most people never come close. They hit their mental limit first. One of the best examples of this is Roger Bannister, the first man to ever break 4 minutes in the 1-mile run. He was told by doctors and coaches that it was a physical impossibility to break the 4-minute-mile. His heart would explode or something like that.

Roger Bannister's perceived limits were much greater than the doctors and coaches perceived limits and it turns out he was right! Weeks after he broke the 4-minute-mile someone else did too and now it seems every year there are high school kids trying to break 4-minutes in the mile. It would have been much less exciting if Roger decided to believe in an early limit on what was possible for him. Not that we need to break a world record but living in a world of potential improvement is much more fun than living in a world of early limitation.

Comparing yourself to others:
Don't compare yourself to others unless it is just for inspiration. When you look at someone who has done anything better than you there are two reactions you can have. One is to feel uncomfortable and inadequate with ourselves so we make excuses for why they have it easier. We try to pull them down or downplay their achievement so we feel better about where we are. I could easily try to come up with reasons why this 10-year-old girl beat me. But that gets me nowhere fast. The fact is she did. I bet she worked harder on that than I did!

The other option we have is to be inspired by them and develop a hunger/desire to get to the place they are at. This is the positive action and the better choice. Have you ever seen someone you know buy a bigger house and a mutual friend starts saying things like "They are lucky they can do that, some of us don't have that kind of money." Or "They work too much they probably have no time for their kids." Or "There are so many charities they could have donated to instead." This person is trying to pull others down so they don't feel bad about their house.

If someone out earns you...
> ...don't say "they cheated their way there"

If someone beats you in a race...
> ...don't say "they are younger than me"

If someone is skinnier than you...
> ...don't say "they are blessed with a fast metabolism"

This downplays the hard work they have put in to be where they are AND you have decreased your hope for growth and betterment. Instead lets say "they worked hard to get there." "I'd like to ask them how they got to that awesome level, maybe I can learn something and get better!"

Being better than someone else
And
Being worse than someone else
Are two sides to the same broken coin.

Some people think being humble is thinking you are less than or worse than other people. That is not humility. If you think you are worse than other people you are just as bad off as the person who thinks they are better than others. We know the problem with thinking we are better than others is not good. Looking down on others turns us into a jerk. We are certainly very limited in our compassion and understanding. If you can be worse than other people then you can also be better than other people. If someone is better than you because they make more money then that means someone who makes less money is worse than you. If someone is better than you because they have great physical abilities that means someone with less physical abilities is worse than you.

At the risk of sounding too much like a hippy or overly spiritual, we are all on this crazy ride together with different experiences and different genes but all of us are valuable just as we are. When you have compassion and understanding for the people around you (including the jerks) you will have more compassion and understanding for yourself. If you rant about other people's actions like they are idiots you will have more times that you feel like an idiot. Not the path to happiness and contentment for sure!

Focusing on the limits:
The final way to be unhappy is to focus on all the things you can't do right now instead of all you can. I see this a lot when people have arthritis or an injury but it also shows up when someone hasn't worked out in decades and comes into a group of people who have been working out 5 days a week for months or some cases years! We tend to fixate on the things we cannot do. Why are the stories of the people with missing limbs that go on with life and achieve so inspiring? I think it's because they got over the focusing on limitations and instead focused on what they can do. We all have limitations. We are all disabled in certain ways. If we can focus on improvement and ability we will be much happier in the process. If you have bone on bone knees there are certain exercises you absolutely SHOULD NOT DO! If you throw a pity party constantly you won't make any improvements because you are most likely going to give up because you can't do everything. Even someone with no knees can have hope! They can improve! Focus on the good you CAN DO even if it feels like such a small area to start off with.

30 – The Key to Unhappiness

For the person joining a gym where people have been there for years, you won't be able to do what they can do right away. If you set the goal at beating or matching someone who has been at it for years you are more likely to give up because it is going to take too long before you see that happen. Instead look for improvement. The first week of exercise you won't see much if any. You'll mostly feel sore and tired. (The second week gets better.) Remind yourself that although you are not the strongest or the fastest you are getting stronger and faster than you were last week when you didn't workout at all. Be patient and focus on the good you are doing. You will improve. And you can enjoy the process that much more.

We are all capable of more than we think. With training and practice I too might be able to out run that 10-year-old. If my value comes from that though it's coming from the wrong place. So we need to believe we are capable of amazing things, see others as inspiration not as better than us, and focus on the good we are doing however small it is right now. If we can do that we will find exercise and life in general to be a happier more successful ride.

31
Realize U Ain't Perfect

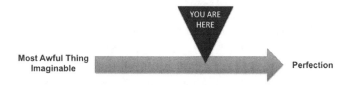

Most Awful Thing Imaginable ————————▶ Perfection

YOU ARE HERE

I want to yell, "FREEEEEEDOM!", like Mel Gibson's character in "Braveheart." I'm going to release you from the bondage of perfectionism. Well, help start the process anyway! Perfectionism is a prison that prevents you from taking action and doesn't allow you to see opportunities.

Two Damaging Phrases of Perfectionism:
- "I'm doing everything right, why is my weight not down?"
- "Once I'm through with this busy season then I'll make this change."

What's the problem with these statements? I've said both of these. (I can speak about the dangers of perfectionism because I'm still a recovering perfectionist, with relapses occasionally).

"I'm doing everything right"…

I often halfway joke with clients about this one. I've never had a day when I did everything right. I'm not sure I've had a minute where I did everything right. When this

148

statement is used we are probably doing a lot of this right and more right than we feel we ever have before. However, there is the nasty prison this statement builds: If you are stuck and you are doing everything right then there is no way out! But, that's not so bad since you are already perfect. :o)

What can you improve on? What can you learn? Nothing! Because you are already doing everything right! Now I realize this statement is used as an exaggeration. Like, "I've told you a million times not to do that!" We don't really mean a million times, we just mean a lot of times. I believe in the power of words to either shut down our brains or fire them up. "I did everything right", shuts down our creative imagination, while a statement like, "I've been working hard is there something I'm missing?", begins to open up our creative part of our brain. It allows the brain to run.

When someone says this perfection statement, "I'm doing everything right." I cannot help them without delicately calling them a liar. People don't like being called liars. This statement is also usually a sign that the person has already given up. It can be helpful to think of yourself like the little irish football player in the movie "Rudy." You've been knocked down for the 100th time that day and as you lie there on your back or on your face you have a choice to make. Quit and deal with the consequences of failure or get back up and try again.

Sometimes you need a little encouragement and some new ideas.

My daughter Anna was a perfect example of this. I took her to a bounce house place for a Daddy and Daughter date. There is a gigantic scaffolding type structure in there that's ½ fun house and ½ maze. They discourage parents from playing on the equipment so I had to send her up there all alone. She was 3 ½ years old. She decided she wanted to climb the slide that was way up there. She started climbing and made it just over halfway where the slide gets steeper and her slippery socks wouldn't let her go any farther. She dropped to her knees flopped to her stomach and slid down. She tried again and again and again. Some kids were coming down and she moved out of the way then tried again. It was clear that just trying harder at the same thing wasn't working to daddy. I was in love with her determination though.

I got her attention and told her to pull her long pants up above her knees. (I would have told her to take her socks off but then they'd have been lost 3 stories up). She needed better grip and when she dropped to her knees at the halfway point she would get it. She pulled her pants up and tried again. She climbed and reached the halfway point and the socks started to slip. She dropped to her knees and realized she was stuck there a little. She began to climb. The slide kept getting steeper. It was hard. I still wasn't sure that would be enough to get her to the top. She grunted and worked and pulled herself up on the platform. I was a ninny and started jumping around with tears coming to my eyes full of daddy pride. She pulled her pant legs back down and got back to playing. She climbed that slide 5-7 more times that day. Every time pulling her pant legs up before climbing. She made it every time even when she was getting a little tired.

I want to encourage you to get back up and try again like my determined daughter. But don't try it the exact same way. The definition of insanity is doing the same action over and over and expecting a different result. Get up and try it a little differently. My job as a trainer is to help people find a new focus every time they get knocked down. I encourage them to try again. That there is something they still haven't tried or a different men, state to try again with. I don't know your individual challenge since you aren't talking back to me so if you are feeling like giving up, I will ask you this question, "Assuming you are not perfect what is something new you can try this time?" (Hopefully other sections of this book will give you a ton of ideas)

"Once I'm through with this busy"…

This is perfectionism at work. Sometimes we just think of this as busyism. The core concept at play in this statement is that somehow in the future there will be a time when you aren't very busy and have tons of time to do _____ (whatever it is you want to achieve). I've done this one myself (still do). There is no perfect time. Why does our car always break down at the worst time? Because it's nearly always a bad time to have your car break down!

There will be no perfect season. There is some good you can do today. We can change our past, present, and future. We do this based on what we do today. Actions today will bring about a different future for us and today will become our past. Every spiritual teaching, I'm not even talking just Christianity here, has a strong push to live our lives today. We don't know what the future holds for us.

We can take action now. If we have time to eat we can eat healthier. Which by the way will give us more energy, mental clarity, and boost our immune system. All good things to have when you are in a tight spot in life. If you have time to shower you have time to do 1 minute of exercise before. Make small steps. The work you do now is like investing in your retirement fund. The more you invest and the earlier you invest the "fund" gets exponentially better. Don't wait for the perfect time. It's not coming. Do something imperfect but in a positive direction today and experience FREEEEEDOOOMMM!!!

Conclusion: Weight Loss is a Guided Missile Not a Magic Bullet

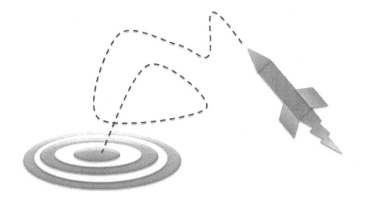

Ready, Aim, FIRE! This is the process for firing a bullet. Once the bullet leaves the gun you no longer have any influence over it so you better take your time and AIM that thing! Weight loss is not like this. Weight loss is more like a guided missile than a bullet. We make course corrections on the way (and perhaps like a missile we are a bit farther from our goal).

Why is this important to me that you understand this distinction?

1.) We spend too much time aiming. We try to get the "perfect" plan together before we get started. The truth is we will always have incomplete knowledge as we set out to do something or achieve something of worth. We will use up too much precious time waiting for every little detail. If you are like me you can name a few things that you KNOW you can do right now that would make you healthier. It ain't a perfect knowing but it's enough to push the launch button. George S. Patton is quoted as saying. "A good plan, violently executed now, is better than a perfect plan next week."

2.) We hope for some kind of magic one size fits all answer. It isn't coming. One size fits most is available, but there are plenty of things that are going to work for someone else but they aren't going to work for you. Don't wait for the magic pill or secret recipe. Fire!

3.) Momentum is the key. I often think about this in my spiritual life. God cannot steer me if I'm not moving! I have this happen with training clients, they want some advice on what to do with their nutrition but they aren't keeping records so I have nothing to tell them except the basics. When a missile is fired it is constantly sending signals to mission control (or home base) about where it is and what it is doing. Then mission control sends signals back to move slightly to the right or left, up or down. Thousands of small course corrections on its way to the target. Just like in weight loss and health, the course corrections get smaller and smaller the closer to the target you get.

In Steven Covey's book "7 Habits of Highly Effective People" one of the big points he makes is about education and action balance. He calls it Production Vs. Production Capability. You do need to balance these two. Production (or action) is the go getter. Up and at 'em. Charging ahead. Many of us are missing this part or this part is too weak so we sit and wait for more information when we have enough to get started. Production

Conclusion

Capability (or Education) is the learning and trying to find the "right" way. Both are important. Without action we are dead in the water and without education we could be running full speed in the opposite direction. The best formula for weight loss and health success is pick up enough info to get started and take moments to check progress, review, and seek new ideas as you charge ahead.

But...

This is where weight loss and health is nothing like a missile. A missile has a target it hits the target blows up and is finished. If WE hit the target and stop all our work we back slide. Most of us have had first hand experience at this. It's heartbreaking and it takes awhile (sometimes years) to get the gumption to try again.

As we work to gain momentum, take action, and constantly course correct we need to embrace reality as it is. We will always need to use some effort in this area. Just like getting a car moving by pushing it. Oh boy is it tough to get started! Once it's rolling it only takes a little consistent effort to keep it rolling. Unless you hit one of those hills of life. Then you might need to let others come in and push with you. Please don't just read this book. DO SOMETHING! Fire! Then aim and course correct!

Extra Resources

Quick Start Guide
10 Minute Resistance Workout
10 Minute Cardio Workout
Post Workout Stretch Routine
Craving Management (Stop Cravings)
Jeremy's Story
Sarah's Story
Anna's Story

Quick Start Guide

If you are reading the quick start guide I'm guessing you want to see results fast. Results are where motivation comes from. So getting it started fast is a great idea. Just remember your results won't last unless you fortify them with the rest of the information in this book. With that said, I would tell you to focus on 3 things to get some quick wins.

#1 - Food Journal - Sure it's not magic but it works better than any supplement or weight loss pill ever invented. Food Journal for a week weighing everything on a digital food scale and try not to have a positive result. To get access to our software visit www.talltrainer.com/31lessons

#2 - Exercise 5 days a week - Monday - Friday like it's your job. The consistency will bring massive results. If you don't know what to do and you don't have much history with sticking to a program try these two 10 minute workouts. One Minute Each Exercise and 10 Exercises. Alternate days with these two workouts to get a quick start. If you are way out of the exercise routine I would just do one round per day the first week. The second week you could add in a second round after a minute or two rest and water break. You can do up to 4 rounds of these workouts, but if you are tight on time a regular pattern of 10 minutes per day beats an irregular 40+ minutes per day.

Exercise Pictures and Descriptions in the next sections…

#3 – Invite someone to join you. You will go harder and stick with it longer with someone else on your team.

Fitness in Real Life

If you REALLY want to be successful you need to build your support structure.

10 Minute No Equipment Resistance Workout

Workout Video Available At:
www.talltrainer.com/31lessonsbook

This workout is more for your muscles but will still get your heart rate up and have you sweating. There are thousands of exercises with equipment but I wanted to remove any excuse for getting started I possibly could. This is a well balanced no equipment workout that you could do to improve your health. Keep in mind not all exercises are good for all people. This workout is great if done correctly and by someone without a lot of prior injuries. Study the pictures, read the descriptions, go to the website and watch the videos to make sure you do it safely and effectively. If you feel joint pain or very specific muscle pain about the size you could cover with your thumb stop the exercise because something is wrong. When in doubt get face to face with an exercise professional.

One minute each exercise then move on to the next. If you cannot keep going on the exercise, pause, then try some more if you still have time left in your minute. As you get stronger you will need fewer and fewer rest breaks.

1.) Jog in Place
2.) YTI
3.) Split Squat
4.) Split Squat

Fitness in Real Life

5.) Push-Ups
6.) Punch the Air
7.) Scissor ABS
8.) Plank
9.) Ice Skaters
10.) Sprint in Place

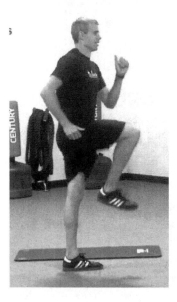

1.) Jog in Place – (warm-up) Starting off the workout in a more warm-up type fashion will make this safer. If jogging hurts your knees or feels too jarring you can march in place. Moving the arms and legs, standing up straight, and landing quietly are a couple good reminders.

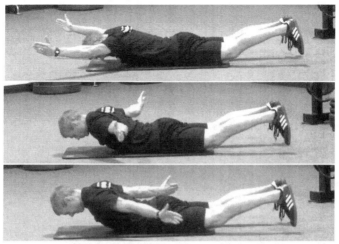

2.) YTI – (for the shoulders and upper back) – Lay on your stomach on the ground. Pull your abdominals (stomach) in and keep your shoulders away from your ears. The 'Y' is done with the arms overhead with thumbs pointing to the ceiling the whole time. Make sure you look at the floor while doing this or your neck will get too much work. Pause and hold the 'Y' position for a couple seconds reminding yourself to look down and slide your shoulders away from the years. Then move to the 'T' position arms out at your sides. It's like you are pretending to be an airplane. The 'I' position for this version is going to be hands down by your hips still rotating hands outward to still kind of have the thumbs up. Squeeze shoulders away from the ears again. Then move back to the 'Y' position and continue until your minute is up. To make it tougher try to raise your arms higher off the ground but don't tighten your neck muscles, don't let your shoulders slide up to your ears, and don't arch your back (keep abs and butt tight). You should feel this in your shoulders and between your shoulder blades. Your arms will get pretty heavy during that minute.

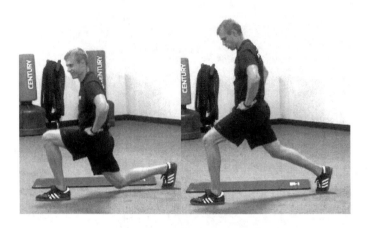

3.) and 4.) Split Squat – (for the legs) One Minute on one side and one minute on the other. This is a pretty challenging exercise even without any weights to hold. Standing slide one foot back behind you or step one foot forward so you find yourself in a lunge position. If you aren't sure how to get that you can kneel for a moment then tuck your toes up on the back foot and push yourself away from the ground. We are trying to put most of our body weight on our front leg as we do this exercise. Weight on the heel of the front foot and slightly more pressure on the outside edge (pinky toe side) of the foot. If you are new to this exercise you may not be able to go down very far yet. Don't push it too hard trying to get low because you need to give your body time to get more flexible too. On day one don't go too hard because this exercise can make you sore. If you can't do any more you can rest until the minute is up then try the other side. Front knee should stay over the front ankle and not move too much. The knee also won't go fully straight on this exercise. If it does you will be putting too much pressure on your knees. You should feel this exercise in your thighs, butt, and calves. Maintain good upper body posture throughout with the addition of a slight lean forward to keep weight on the front leg. Shoulders away from ears, chest out, and back straight.

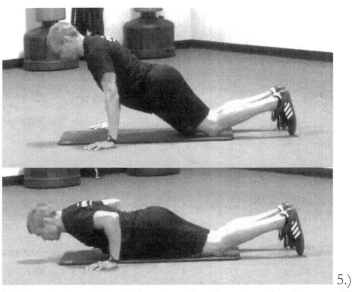

5.)
Push-Ups – (chest and arms) An exercise classic yet still done wrong about 90% of the time. Many people don't have the strength for this exercise yet so they could do this on the stairs or a counter top. Posture is more important than range of motion which is more important than doing the exercise on the ground from toes (hard version). If you think you are pretty strong please still start from knees instead of toes. Setup with shoulders away from the ears, chin pulled back, and head out in front of hands. Then lower yourself down and push yourself back up. Make sure you do not strain your neck by trying to reach your head to the floor. Poor push-ups done regularly can really hurt your shoulders, great push-ups on the other hand can be very helpful for your shoulders. If you don't think you are doing it right it would be better in the long run to skip this exercise than do it wrong.

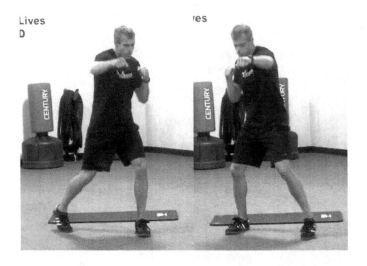

6.) Punch the Air – (more for heart rate) This exercise is added to get your heart rate up OR so you can do it slowly and actively recover from the exercises you have already done. You choose based on how you are feeling. While standing turn your foot on the floor and punch your fist out in front of you then turn back and rotate the other foot out and throw the other fist. This rotation on the feet is a great habit to learn so we are better at taking care of our knees and back. Try to exhale with each punch. Make sure your elbow doesn't lock out straight a slight slight bend in the elbow on the punch out will be better for the joint. The hand that isn't punching will be by your face like you are talking on the phone and then punches out from there.

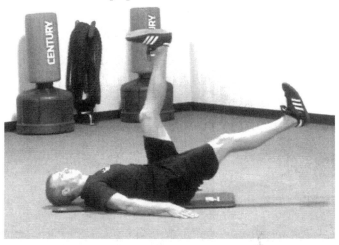

7.) Scissor ABS – (abdominals) Lay on your back and pull your stomach muscles in. Lift both feet off the ground. Raise one leg up as high and as towards you as you can while keeping it straight. Then switch legs. Try to keep the lower back pressing towards the ground and avoid arching your back. Keep a slight bend in your legs so you don't overwork your hip flexor instead of your abs. Keep the neck relaxed as you do this one sometimes it tries to help. You should feel this in your abdominals/stomach area. If you feel it in your back tighten your abs more or make the range of motion smaller.

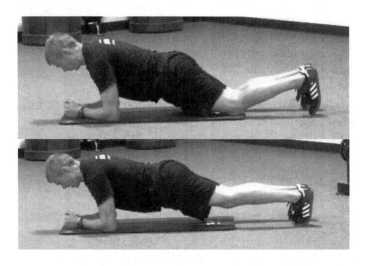

8.) Plank – (abdominals again) A little set of back to back abdominal exercises to make sure you get them well. Facing the floor prop yourself up on your elbows and knees with your hips low to start. If a minute of that is too easy then try elbows and toes. Make sure you have good upper body posture chest out, shoulders away from the ears, eyes looking at floor or hands. Try a slight bend in the knees to keep the work in the lower abdominals. Consciously tighten the abdominals. You might feel this in your shoulders some so make sure you've got good posture. You should certainly feel it in your abdominals. If you feel lower back try to tighten the abs more.

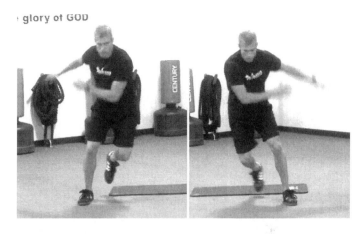

9.) Ice Skaters – (legs and heart rate) Standing up you are going to hop or step from one leg to the other. The bigger the hop/step the more it will get your heart rate up. It looks like you are an Olympic Speed Skater. You should feel this in your heart and lungs and hips and calves.

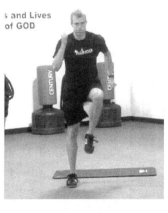

10.) Sprint in Place – (heart rate and metabolism boost) Finishing with some cardio will get the metabolism fired up a little. I suppose there doesn't need to be as much information. It's running but in place. If your knees or feet can't handle the work then leave your feet still and just pump your arms like you are running (you can still get pretty tired this way). Shoulders away from ears, chest out, good posture. Make sure you aren't stomping. Fast is good to get heart rate up but also large movements (like lifting knees and pumping arms bigger) get the heart rate up as well. Try to finish in a way that makes it take a minute to catch your breath.

I hope you enjoy this workout and it can remove obstacles like time and equipment since it only takes 10 minutes and no equipment. Consistency matters. Do this regularly and you will notice the benefits continue to build. I recommend finding someone to workout with and play some good music. You'll do it more often that way. If you can't figure out what you are supposed to do from the pictures and the description make sure you check out the video I made for you at www.talltrainer.com/31lessonsbook.

10 Minute No Equipment Cardio

Workout Video Available At:
www.talltrainer.com/31lessonsbook

Here is a workout for your very own living room with no equipment. Of course you could do this outside, in a hotel room, or even in a gym as well. You could probably even do it in a jail cell but hopefully not have to! The idea is to remove obstacles to exercise. This removes location as an excuse (you don't have to travel). It removes equipment as an excuse (you don't need any). And I think it removes time as an excuse as well (if you don't have 10 minutes for exercise you clearly don't WANT to have 10 minutes available).

In the video on the books resource page (www.talltrainer.com/31lessonsbook) I will demonstrate these exercises and show you options in case you have an injury. If you feel joint pain or very specific muscle pain you should stop right away. Something isn't working right. This workout may not work for everyone but it should work for most people. I encourage you not to do this workout alone. It's more fun and you will be held accountable and work harder with someone else plus if you have an issue someone would be there to help you.

1.) Jumping Jacks
2.) Tap Back Reach Ups
3.) Mountain Climbers
4.) Shuffle Punch
5.) Tantrum
6.) Repeater Knees 10x each

Fitness in Real Life

7.) Burpees
8.) Duck Jabs
9.) Alternating Kicks
10.) Drum Roll

One minute each exercise then move on to the next. If you cannot keep going on the exercise, pause, then try some more if you still have time left in your minute. As you get stronger you will need fewer and fewer rest breaks.

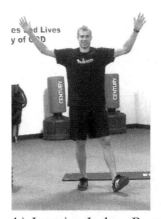 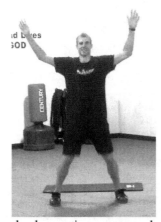

1.) Jumping Jacks - Pretty standard exercise you may have seen. Make sure arms stay fairly straight and hands don't go above head level. Those are two common mistakes on this exercise. You can do it with a hop or just tap one heel to the side for a 1/2 jumping jack with no impact. The pattern of movement is jump feet apart or tap out to the side while moving the arms up. Then jump or tap feet together as you bring your arms down. (Make sure your knees don't cave in on the landing if you are hoping).

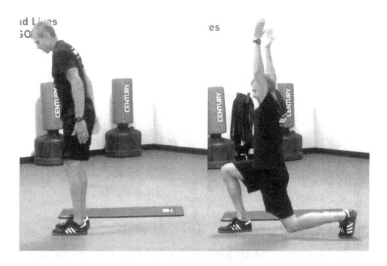

2.) Tap Back Reach Ups - While standing slide one foot back into a lunge while reaching the arms overhead. Step back forward while bringing arms down and repeat this with the other leg. Step farther back and sink lower for additional challenge. These first two exercises are intended to be more warm-up like but still get the heart rate up. Keep the abs tight when reaching overhead and make sure you have more weight on your front foot than your back foot. More specifically try to have your weight on the heel and outside edge (pinky toes side) of the front leg. This will keep your knee lined up properly.

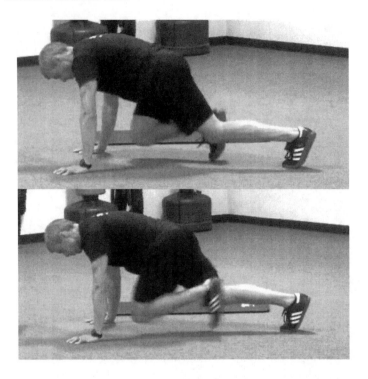

3.) Mountain Climbers – Start off facing the floor in a push-up type position on hands and toes. (You can do this on a sturdy coffee table or the couch to make it a little easier on the arms). Bring one foot in towards the hands and tap the foot on the ground. Bring it back and then bring the other foot in and tap. Repeat this possibly adding A LOT of speed once you get the pattern. Make sure you aren't pushing off with the foot that is closer to the hands because it will put bad pressure on your knee in that position and make your body hop up and down more than needed. Try to keep the body relatively still to get the core working more. This one should get the heart rate up pretty well.

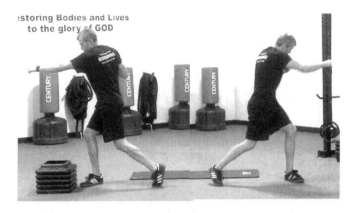

4.) Shuffle Punch – Shuffle your feet to the left 2-3x then turn to the left making sure to pivot and turn your right foot with you and punch your right fist to the left. Then shuffle right 2-3x turn right, pivot right, and punch left hand to the right. Repeat picking up speed as you feel more confident. Make sure you lift your feet as you shuffle or you might trip! :o)

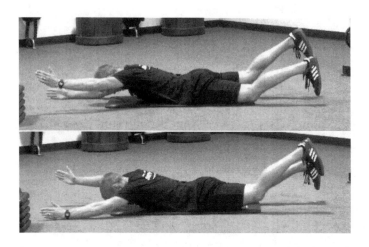

5.) Tantrum – Lying on your stomach tighten your abs and lift your arms and legs slightly off the ground. Tighten your butt to lift your legs. Then raise one hand higher along with the opposite leg. (Ex. Left arm and right leg). Then switch which arm and leg are raised. Keep switching back and forth so it looks like you are throwing a tantrum on the floor. Look down so you don't tighten your neck too much. If you feel your lower back too much (especially if it's sharp) try tightening the abs more and not raising arms and legs as high off the ground. You should feel this in the back of the shoulders, butt, and some warming in your lower back and abs. If it's tough to breathe there most likely isn't anything wrong with you, it's tough to breathe from this position.

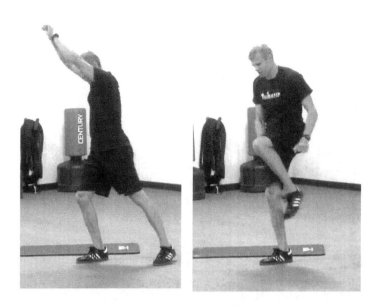

6.) Repeater Knees 10x each – Standing up tap one foot about 12 inches behind the other then bring that knee up to hip height (or higher if you can do that with your back straight). Repeat 10x then switch to the other leg and do the same. When the foot is on the ground raise your arms up into the air. As you bring the knee up bring the arms down like you are grabbing a stick out of a tree and snapping it on your knee. Don't push off the ground too hard with the foot in the back because it might get your calves a little too much. Keep your back straight the whole time.

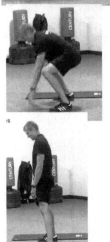

7.) Burpees – Start from a standing position. We try for feet a little wide at the start so the movement works more like a squat (easier on the knees). Squat down and touch the floor. If you can't do this while keeping your back straight then use a stair, coffee table, or some other elevated surface. Once you have your hands on the ground you can either step your feet back one at a time or jump them both back simultaneously. Then reverse the process. Jump or step the feet forward (and slightly wide). Then stand back up (some people jump up from there). Whatever way you choose to do Burpees make sure your body feels able to do it correctly.

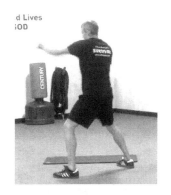
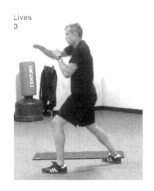
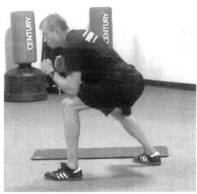

8.) Duck Jabs – Two punches one duck. Standing with feet in a squat stance or a partial lunge stance (slight front and back stance), Throw two punches at an imaginary opponent. Then duck by bending the legs and tipping forward at the hips slightly. (Do not bend your back here!) Your head will lower like you are ducking under and dodging an opponents punches. Repeat. Punch, Punch, Duck, Punch, Punch, Duck.

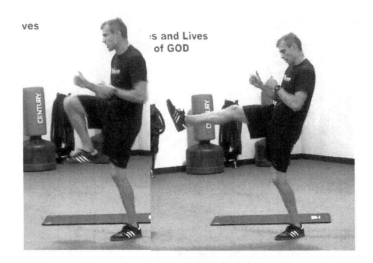

9.) Alternating Kicks – Standing lift one knee up then push foot out straightening the knee. Re-bend the knee while keeping it lifted (pull the foot back). Lower the knee setting the foot on the floor. Repeat on the other leg. Keep abs tight and lean back slightly on the kick. Start with lower kicks until your flexibility improves.

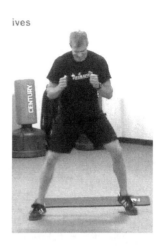
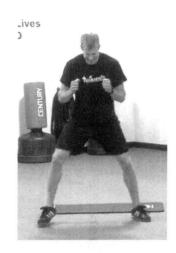

10.) Drum Roll – Standing with wide stance (feet about 2-3 feet apart). Alternate lifting a foot of the ground slightly and bring it back down. It's like a wide and fast jog in place. This is done super fast so it seems more like you are vibrating or playing the floor like a drum. This is not a good exercise if someone is sleeping in a room below you. It makes a great finishing exercise because you can get a big burn and huff and puff with low risk of injury.

I will suggest again to visit the page:
www.talltrainer.com/31lessonsbook
There you can see a video description of the workout to make sure you understood the directions correctly. If you have pain in a joint or a sharp pain in a muscle stop right away (do not push through) something is not working right. I hope you find this workout a great fall back when you don't have equipment available and you don't have much time. No reason not to get a workout most days of the week even if you are busy!

Basic Stretching Routine:

This is the set of stretches we finish every workout with. We do the same stretches everyday because we want to develop a habit of stretching at the end of workouts for our clients. It becomes a memorized pattern over time. Anything you do daily has incredible power over time. One day then never again has very little influence, but everyday starts to compound. A daily habit of stretching is a GREAT habit to develop. I'm convinced our daily stretching is one reason why people feel so good in our program!

Hold each stretch for 30 seconds each. (Total of 8 minutes of stretching)

1. **Knee Pull-in**
2. **Ankle over knee**
3. **Overhead Triceps**
4. **Hamstring**
5. **Hip Flexor**
6. **Quadriceps**
7. **Calf Stretch**
8. **Chest Stretch**

Details…

Basic Stretching Routine

1. Knee Pull-in (hip stretch)

This is one of my favorite stretches because of my own personal low back injury. It is a stretch that helps lay the foundation of movement with hips without movement in the low back. If you have spent any time sitting you may compromise your back position because your hips are tight. You might not feel this stretch much but if you do it will be in the groin (inner thigh) or Hip/Butt/Upper Hamstring area.

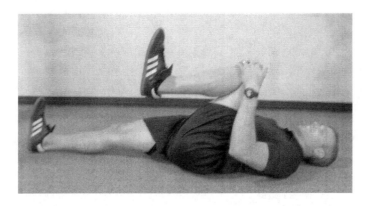

HOW TO - Lay on your back on the floor. Lay one leg flat on the ground and bend your other leg and pull it towards you. Try to keep an arch in your lower back as you do this. The harder you pull the more you will notice you lower back wants to push into the floor. Imagine you are trying to keep a slight arch like a tunnel for a tiny ant train to drive under. Keep your shoulders away from your ears, chest out, and head on the floor as you do this stretch. Some people won't get much stretch and some won't be able to get their leg very close to them.

2. Ankle over knee (more hip stretch)

This is another in the same family of stretches for the hip. This helps with rotational ability at the hip. External rotation specifically. Known by some as a Pirformis stretch I usually just tell people they should feel it in their butt. You might feel it in the groin also.

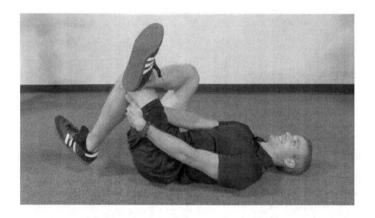

HOW TO - Still laying on your back cross one ankle over the opposite knee. Grab your bottom leg (non-crossed leg) Reach around the outside of the leg with one arm and through the window you just made with your other arm. While trying to keep your head on the ground and your tailbone on the ground pull the legs towards you. Try to keep an arch in the back like the last stretch. Once you have this try to flex your toes back towards your knee on the leg that is crossed over. It will keep the knee more stable and will move some of the twisting force out of the knee and into the hip. (There are other options if you cannot reach your leg because the muscles are so tight)

3. Overhead Triceps (Armpit Stretch)

This is a great stretch for those who have poor posture or are seated much of the day. Tightness in this area can lead to shoulder joint pain and inability to reach things on the top shelf. If your shoulders are already beat up start this stretch carefully.

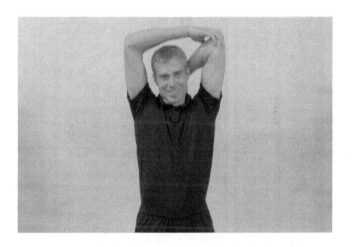

HOW TO - Standing up reach one arm behind you like you are patting yourself on the back. Try to get the hand to touch the shoulder on the same side. Use the non-stretching arm to touch the elbow and help lift and open the shoulder. Try to keep your head in a comfortable position (good posture). This stretch should be felt on the back of the arm (triceps) and down the outside of the armpit (lats). To get more stretch think about pointing the elbow at the ceiling.

4. Hamstring (Back of the Leg Stretch)

I don't meet to many people who don't have tight hamstrings because on average we sit too long everyday. Tight hamstrings can cause an amazing amount of back pain.

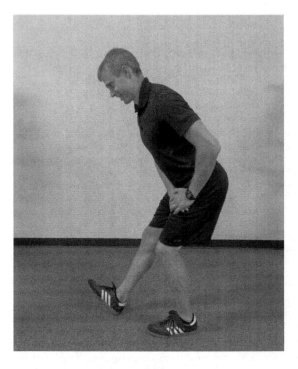

HOW TO - Standing kick one foot out in front of you about 12 inches and place your heel on the floor. Keep this leg straight, stick your chest out and tailbone out (to keep the back straight). Imagine you have a dial at your hips and you turn that dial to tip forward more so the movement comes from the hips and not bending the back. For a little extra fun you can add in some calf stretch by pulling your toes back towards you. It's not a bad idea but it won't feel comfortable. You should feel this stretch from your butt all the way to your heel.

Basic Stretching Routine

5. Hip Flexor (front of hip stretch)

When you sit your hip also gets very tight in the front as it is stuck in a bent position. When you stand up this muscle sometimes doesn't fully loosen so you end up with bad posture and a bigger than necessary arch in your back. This again can cause back and knee pain.

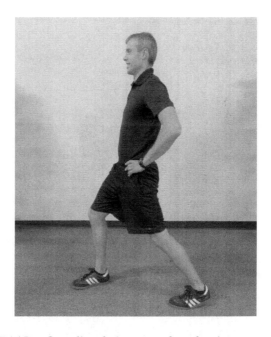

HOW TO - Standing bring one foot back so you are in a partial lunge stance. Pretend like you have a cool belt buckle on and you want to see it and tip your hips up towards you so you can see the imaginary belt buckle. This is called posteriorly rotating your pelvis. Then press back leg behind you as you bend the front leg slightly. If you have seen a dog get up from laying down you may have seen a version of this stretch. You should feel the stretch in the front of the hip/thigh on the back leg. If you don't it is most likely you are not rotating your hips up in front.

6. Quadriceps (thigh stretch)

This muscle group again gets tight from sitting. Tightness can cause back, hip, or knee pain. It is also a stretch that I did wrong for many years in sports (and so did everyone else I was copying). It wasn't until I studied some Yoga combined with my understanding of kinesiology that I finally got it. Hopefully I can shorten the learning cycle for you.

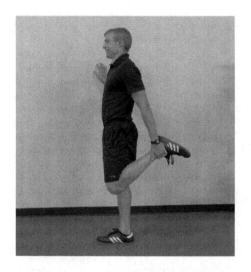

HOW TO - Standing by a wall lift one foot off the ground and grab it by the ankle with the hand from that same side. (Left hand grabs left ankle). What you need to do next is point your knee down at the ground. It will have a tendency to point forward slightly. Keep the abdominals tight as this stretch makes people arch their back instead of stretch the thigh sometimes. So knee points down, abs in tight, and imagine you are trying to push your hips in front of that knee. At some point before your foot touches the back of your head you should feel a stretch. You should feel it all along the top of the thigh and in the front of the hip. This is also a great hip flexor stretch too.

Basic Stretching Routine

7. Calf (back of lower leg stretch)

Sitting and walking do not afford much stretch for the calf muscle and shoes with a higher heel than forefoot don't do much for it either. (Example. of course high heel shoes but also most running shoes are in this same category) Tight calves most directly can hurt the foot or knees. A lot of tendonitis and plantar fasciitis is caused by tight calves.

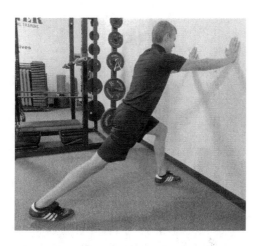

HOW TO - Standing facing a wall or other unmovable surface. Put one foot near the wall and the other foot WAY back. This should have you in a big lunge stance. Put your hands on the wall like you are getting arrested. Make sure you feet are both facing the wall. The back foot will try to turn out. If anything you can turn it in slightly to get a bigger calf stretch. Press into the wall with your hands and push your back heel towards the ground. If you aren't feeling the stretch in the back of the leg between ankle and knee then bend the leg closest to the wall. That should get you a better stretching angle. This stretch can also be done with a slightly bent back leg to get more towards your achillies tendon (by your heel).

8. Chest Stretch

When you slouch all day your upper back muscles get weak and your chest gets tightened up because you just don't ask it to ever stretch. This is a big culprit for shoulder injuries specifically the rotator cuff.

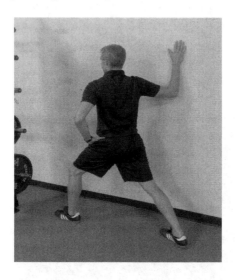

HOW TO - Standing near a wall place your arm on the wall with hand pointing to ceiling and your elbow about shoulder height. Step forward with your outside foot (if left arm is on the wall you step forward with your right foot). Shrug your shoulders away from your ears and stick your chest out. This will get your shoulder in the right position to stretch. Then turn away from the arm on the wall slightly. If you turn a lot you will be fooling yourself into thinking you are flexible. It is a very small turn. I have found this stretch works best when the feet are farther apart. You should feel this stretch in your chest of course not in your shoulder joint and certainly not down your arm.) The more you feel this stretch towards the middle of your chest the better and healthier the stretch is for you.

Basic Stretching Routine
One last word on these stretches:

When in doubt with any of these stretches please use caution and get coaching. Anything you do consistently has great power. If you do it consistently wrong it can cause problems. If done consistently right it solves and prevents problems.

Jeremy's Fitness and Health Story

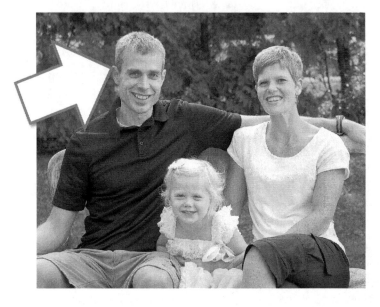

This is of course an on going journey but I'll share how I got to where I am...

The best place to start is High School. That's when the interest in exercise really began. I was a below average athlete. You can tell your ranking pretty fast by how soon you get picked for a team in gym class. I wasn't last but I was near the bottom of the roster. I was growing rapidly to my now 6'3" height. My muscles weren't exactly keeping up. It seemed like I got tighter, weaker, and slower as I grew taller. One point of pride I always had was back in elementary school I was one of the first kids who could climb the rope. This was only due to my near constant desire to climb trees as a kid. Other than that brief moment my gym class performance was lack luster.

I believe that affinity for tree climbing was a precursor to my enjoyment of pole-vaulting. I started pole-vaulting in 9th grade. Basically I didn't like finishing second to last in the 2 mile (I tried really hard not to be last!). Running 8 laps on the track was like boring torture especially as I looped around and found the pole-vaulters lying on the mats for the majority of practice. I decided I wanted in on that! (Notice I chose my event based on how much nap time I might get). I started working out with the pole-vaulters but still had to run the 2-mile at meets. It wasn't until 10th grade that I got to focus more on pole vault. I loved it right away and not just the laying on the mats part. Hard work equaled more flying and landing on soft mats. Beginning my 10th grade season as a pole-vaulter I was one of three sophomore pole-vaulters without any more experienced upper classmen. I feel it was a God type blessing because it gave me and my sophmore teammates a chance that most athletes never get. We got to compete as the top 3 vaulters even though we weren't very good yet. Through repetition and stubbornness we all got better. It was then I realized I wanted to get stronger and faster so I could do better. I just didn't want to get tired, out of breath, or sore. Hummmm? I was going to have to get over that. To know how bad it was we were supposed to run a 2-lap warm-up at the start of practice. I would either run a ½ lap and uncover the mats or just hide behind them and join in for the second lap and do the other ½ of my 1 warm-up lap.

I share this much detail because I want you to know I did not start off with some great love for "the burn" or exercise for exercise sake. I still don't like exercise for exercise sake. If it wasn't for the benefits from exercise I would never do it. But I have learned the benefits can outweigh the effort you put in. In fact there is no other way to feel the strength, health, vitality, energy, and ability without exercise. I fell in love with exercise first. By the time I was a senior on the track team I was out at practice getting my warm-up and first jumps in 30 min before practice even started and I would stay out after practice ended. I even began doing most of my sprint workouts (I still didn't like them, but they were a necessary evil). As I learned about how exercise could help me pole-vault better I got most of my ideas from watching the upperclassmen and generic gym knowledge. No one talked about posture it was just about moving the biggest weight you could in the weight room. I did a lot of things wrong that really ended up catching up with me in college. When I blew my back out training and pole-vaulting it ended my ability to vault and my ability to pick up a pen off the floor. There I was a college athlete about 21 years old with a ruptured L5-S1 disc and shoes that needed to be tied. I remember those months. The doctors said to rest it. So I did for 6 months. I stood in the back of my college classes and lounged in my desk chair (one of the only places I didn't hurt). I could also sit on the couch but only if I had a crazy amount of pillows behind me. I eventually found the one and only position I could sleep in at night that required no less than 4 pillows to create.

What did I get after 6-months of rest? I got weaker. I got depressed. I got no relief from the back pain. I was sick and tired of being sick and tired. I made a contract with myself. "If I'm going to hurt no matter what I do I at least want to be the strongest IN PAIN I could be." So it began. The come back story. It was slow. I stopped taking my daily regiment of Ibuprophen. I would still take it at night before bed but I stopped taking it before classes and definitely stopped taking it before workouts. It made me a more careful exerciser. I had to learn how to use my core to brace my back while working my other body parts.

Jeremy's Health and Fitness Story

I made slow progress, but it was progress. Eventually I was feeling stronger and it scared me to say but my back was feeling a little bit better too.

I tried vaulting again but the pain intensified the harder I tried. With many tears I gave it up. It's tough to give up the only thing you feel you've ever been good at. Thankfully God had been working in my life before this because during this time I was making nearly straight A's in school (only one B at ACU). I decided I was good at other things too. I was smart and I loved the Exercise Science that I was studying. I realized I was a pretty good coach because of the fact I wasn't a gifted athlete. I knew what it was like to struggle. Great athletes sometimes don't make great coaches as their best advice is, "you just do it." How do you run faster? You just do it? I had learned there was more to it than that. I decided I was either going to Physical Therapy School (All my mistakes had me familiar with the benefit of a good physical therapist to put you back together) or I was going to be a Physical Education and Health teacher and coach sports. I decided to graduate with both options available to me. This meant I got to learn how to teach in the teaching department and I got to learn how the body works from the Exercise Science department. Both were such a blessing and I use both areas everyday. Who knew?

Neither one of these majors were personal training. How did I get there? My Exercise Science Major required an internship while my teaching major required student teaching. I started with the internship in the town the college was in so I could keep my job as a waiter at a Mexican Restaurant to make it through school. My internship was at Hendrick Health Club in Abilene, TX. Another God moment as I could not have planned it better. So I had learned sports conditioning, injuries, and teaching. I was about to learn everything about the health club industry. I joined after they had broken ground on a massive expansion. They were going to double their floor space and add in tons of group exercise programing. Since I was there I got to do it all. Spinning, kickboxing, Step Class, Yoga/Pilates, I even got to teach a hip hop dance class. I got to learn the ins and outs of group exercise as I was simultaneously learning the 1 on 1 personal training field. I could not have planned this better. As I learned all these new things I was applying them to my injured body and learning how to do these things and not hurt myself. As I got stronger and more flexible I got to where I had almost no symptoms of back pain. This is true today. As long as I keep exercising and stretching my back is awesome!

I decided that I wanted to teach people about exercise and how to feel better, get stronger, and be healthier. I wasn't going to be a PE teacher or a Physical Therapist but I was going to get to use everything I knew everyday as a personal trainer. I worked my way into becoming the manager of the personal training department at this amazing gym that changed the direction of my life. It was then I realized that this place was already awesome and I needed to take what I had learned and bring it to somewhere I had never seen it before. And so I brought it back home to Canandaigua, NY. It's been 10 years since then and all I keep doing is learning. Learning from books, clients, and experts how to help people lose weight, eat healthy, and exercise safely for the maximum benefit. Even better still is my wife and daughter who support and inspire me while simultaneously challenging me to be better in other areas besides exercise. Of course this is the shortened version of my story. If you want to know more we would be better off sitting down to lunch sometime. :o)

Sarah's Health and Fitness Story

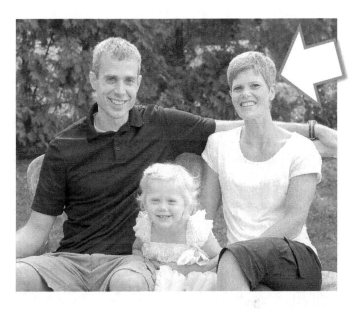

Hi, my name is Sarah and I am a grateful recovering anorexic, bulimic, laxative abuser, excessive exerciser, compulsive overeater and food addict. Needless to say there is a LONG and hairy story that goes with this list that starts from a young age and was a main focus for most of my life. I am no longer ashamed of this past and honestly amazed at the woman I have become.

My back-story:
I was a "solid" kid who was much larger than the other girls in my class. In the 3rd grade I became very aware of my body being bigger. My "dieting" began that year. But I was clueless and I also loved sugar. I steadily gained weight each year using food to cope with events and

emotions I didn't know how to respond to at a young age. THEN came high school! My freshman year in gym class, we all had to stand in a line to get weighed. I had an old hag of a gym teacher who said the numbers out loud as she weighed us. To me she might as well have been announcing this over the loud speaker. As she said the number there were a few that heard it. One boy said "she weighs more than me". *I clearly remember my body trembling, my stomach hitting the floor and literally wanting to DIE! I now LOATHED the scale and it determined my value as a person.* So LONG story still LONG, I attempted to eat healthy starting the summer after my freshman year. By the time gym class rolled around at the start of the next school year I was much smaller (I had lost about 25 pounds over the summer). I could hear my teacher say the weights of my 5 foot nothing classmates and it was still less than me. So I thought I had more work to do. I couldn't think clearly enough to say, "Sarah, you are 7 inches taller than these girls, you should weigh more". **My value was strongly tied to the number on the scale.** I had so many other emotional issues going on (another LONG story) that losing weight became my distraction. By the end of the school year I was 87 pounds and near death. I was still on a mission to lose more. *There was always "5 more" pounds to go.* I still felt "fat" and disgusting at 87 lbs!!

At this point my parents and doctor intervened. I had to start going to a nutrition clinic where I was weighed and my body fat measured weekly. I was a "good patient" if I had gained weight, but I then hated myself. This did not help my loathing of the scale. After a suicide attempt I decided to gain the weight they wanted for me to be "cured". The problem was once I started eating again I had such massive cravings that I had NO idea how to handle. I remember being released from the nutrition clinic as well enough to be on my own. Every one was all happy for me as I was set off on my own. At this point I was a full fledge bulimic and *they had NO idea.* (As an adult in treatment I found out how severe my bulimia was. This wasn't just a little, I ate too much purge, but I will spare you the nasty details. I really shouldn't be alive with my heart, reproductive organs and digestive system functioning well. Praise Jesus!

Then came the college years. I had great *shame* in being bulimic and was wishing to be anorexic again. (OH BROTHER! But truth). After 3 years of starving nearly to death I couldn't stop eating. HOLY CRAVINGS batman!!!!! Let me tell you I ATE and ATE and ATE! Weight started to creep (or not so creep) back to that high school number that told me *"I was bigger than the boys".* So I started running, taking diet pills, and laxatives. These methods helped me to stop the bulimia..oye! What a hot mess I was. At the end of my sophomore year I felt nothing but disgust towards myself, and weight kept continuing to rise. It felt like I had absolutely NO control of my eating. *I remember crying in my dorm room and I called out to God. I clearly heard in my soul "Sarah, there are two paths in life and you are NOT on the right one". It was so moving to me. This was the start of true healing for me. I opened my Bible and everything I read gave me hope and encouragement.* At this point I was at a large state school in Texas and I knew I needed a fresh start. That night I applied to a Christian university and changed my major to health and wellness (was criminal justice). I was determined to learn as much as I could to be healthy and help others.

By the time I graduated college I had stopped the excessive bulimia, diet pills and laxatives but my weight was still climbing. I went to the doctor for a physical and I was nearly 190 pounds. She started to talk to me a little about weight loss. **Now how is that for full circle?** In high school the doctors were demanding I gain weight and now I was being told how to lose weight. This moment on the scale was also life changing for me. There was much shame and embarrassment in this number because I had just graduated with a BS in health and wellness. I knew I had to get this in check or I was going to be even another 100 pounds heavier.

Weight loss was very scary for me. I had fought so hard to overcome severely disordered behaviors and I didn't want to "slip" into old habits. I was determined to do it *slow and steady*. I didn't follow a diet but really tried to listen to my hunger and fullness signals. I became active again doing fun things like roller blading, hiking and riding my bike. This awakened something in me. I enjoyed exercise. It wasn't punishment for something I had eaten but a gift to gain strength and confidence. I ran for fun, not to see how many calories I could burn. I wanted strong arms, not ones that looked like a pencil. I only weighed myself weekly to see where I was. My pants not fitting told me I was going in the right direction.

Over the course of a couple years I was down to a healthy weight and was really finding who I was.

So then life was perfect. I was at my goal weight. Each day was like walking through a field of wildflowers, hearing the birds chirp with the sun beaming on my face. All my troubles and worries were gone. **WRONG!!!** I started weighing myself several times a day in fear that I would wake up one morning and be 190 pounds again. The scale became an obsession. God only knows how many times a day I stepped on that thing. If I was down a pound it was a great day and I would wear cuter clothes. If I were up a couple I would feel like crap and throw on a hat and sweat pants. That day I would vow to be perfect, only eat vegetables and add miles to my run. The next day I was starving and would eat every carb in sight. This usually led to several days of overeating because I was not perfect and felt like garbage about myself. This was the cycle I followed for **YEARS!** I remarkably maintained my weight within 5-10 pounds. Maintained is **not** the correct word. I **BATTLED** my weight within 5-10 pounds. **It was miserable and exhausting**. I was always able to get back down to my "goal weight" quickly but my confidence and personality were deeply affected by this lifestyle!

Somehow I managed to land this super amazing husband and married him quickly before he could really see my crazy☺ I actually gained 20 pounds within the first few months of being married. Once again using food to cope with the many changes that came with marriage (new job, new town, new church, no friends yet, starting a new career path…oh yeah and sharing a living space again). I also became paralyzed with a perfectionist mentality. Here I was married to the "Tall Trainer" and becoming a trainer…I had better be perfect. Turns out when I try to be perfect- I totally rebel and do the opposite. I was slipping into a depression and didn't like the path I was headed down again.

Jeremy is the man I didn't even know how to ask God for. He has inspired me in so many ways. His belief in me, love for me gave me the courage and strength to reach out for help and truly get healing, not just band aide fixes. I had a lot of wounds stuffed deep down inside of me that needed to heal and not be ignored. Lets face it, I pretended I had my past packed away nicely but it was surfacing in many areas of my life. Food was the main way it surfaced.

I changed my outlook on getting "help" and looked at it as an adventure to discover who I was free from food drama. I became a student of myself and started searching with intention for what worked and what didn't. A failure became a lesson and not a failure anymore. I lived life with hope that I WAS going to have a healthy relationship with food and every day I was one day closer to that.

Here's the deal. I know for myself I am not meant to do life alone. It takes a team of people to keep some sort of balance in my life. I need accountability with food, exercise, finances, marriage, smart phone and I am not ashamed of that.

Nutrition wise- I am constantly learning and gaining understanding. I FIGHT to keep foods main focus in my life as 80% fuel for my body and 20% fun. Food has pleasure and enjoyment to me but it is left at that and is not trying to fill some void that food will NEVER fill (for the most part, remember I am perfectly imperfect). I have let my LONG LONG LONG list of food rules GO! Now I make choices on nutrition principles that make me feel and function best. I use the scale as a tool to see if I might not be listening to my body's true hunger needs. (I fluctuate 5-7 pounds and that is completely normal for me). If I start really creeping up it's time to check in with myself.

Fitness Wise-I LOVE being strong. Strong for ME. I don't need to be the strongest, just confident in my strength. I like knowing I could surprise the heck out of someone if they came after my daughter or myself. I like being trained up so I could hop into almost any activity and it wouldn't wreck me for weeks after. I love when my husband chooses me to be on the other end of lifting something heavy out of a room full of people. I love being able to play with my daughter and lift her with ease even at 4 years old. (Yes, I still hold her) I was never an athlete or part of a group sport so exercising in a group fills that void I had always wanted.

Sarah's Health and Fitness Story

Life Wise- My biggest miracle is our daughter Anna Grace. I remember being 16 sitting in the doctors office after a horrible exam. I had not had a period in years and was give steroids to attempt to start it. She told me I most likely would not have children and I was basically 80 years old internally. I know many anorexics and bulimics that this did become a reality and I do not take for granted the miracle of birth that I was so blessed to experience.

I have learned I ALWAYS need to be a student of myself. That I must daily fight for mental, physical and spiritual balance, it does not just happen. That I am worth taking the time to find balance and that I am a better me, wife, mother, trainer and friend when I do that.

This is a beautiful mess of a life ☺

Anna Grace's Story

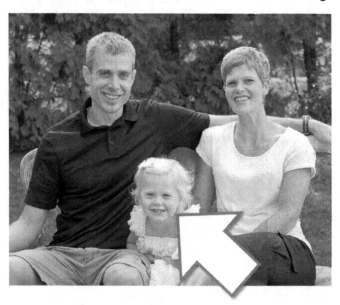

She is still so little and while much of her life is still to be lived there was a few moments that put that in doubt. It all has an amazing outcome that is not nearly the challenge many people have to face, but still different than the cover picture shows. Looking at her you would not know any of this about her. We all have a story that goes way beyond the perfect life that seems captured in pictures.

"They all almost didn't walk out of there." This was the message we got from our doctors and nurses after delivery. It was a pretty common 51 hour labor. Ok so 51 hours isn't so common. I strongly believe if my wife wasn't the physical champ she is we wouldn't have had as nice an outcome. Seriously who can labor for 51 hours? We wanted to do birth as natural as possible but it wasn't progressing fast enough. (Personal opinion) I think too much Pitocin was used and Sarah had a 4-hour contraction. I didn't know how it was different than other labors so no alarms went off for me. When we finally did get to pushing Sarah pushed for 3.5 hours, pretty incredible for someone who has been laboring for that long. Anna's head got stuck. I'm pretty sure Anna's head was bigger than Sarah's hips plus she was coming out sunny side up not over easy.

In an emergency type effort the doctor had to use forceps to free her head. When she came out her head was all sorts of squished (I think more than typical). I remember seeing her for the first time wondering if she was going to make it. Her skin was black, head squished, and she wasn't breathing yet. I just held my breath as the doctors worked to get the baby to breathe while simultaneously trying to sew up my wife who was torn internally and externally. Finally the breath came and with it the tears flowed. One level of relief, she was breathing. Her color came around and Sarah was too weak to hold Anna so I got to hold her. I remember that first snuggle under the blanket with Anna. So amazing and perfect. Then I looked at Sarah as my wife was turning grey-er by the minute. I was reminding myself that Sarah has extra blood during pregnancy for this very reason but as the staff slid around the room in a pool of her blood I wasn't so sure she was going to have enough. I remember getting scared, "I have this cute amazing baby in my arms am I going to be raising her on my own?" They sewed her up and she started to look better.

We had made it.

Everyone was doing well and recovering. It wasn't until a check up a few weeks out that they heard the murmur in Anna's heart at her well child visit. The very next day we had an appointment up at strong in the pediatric cardiac unit for an ECG and meeting with a surgeon. When you get an appointment within 24-hours it makes you nervous. I would say we didn't sleep well that night but we already weren't sleeping well, we had a newborn! The tests came back that she had a medium to large hole in her heart that was causing some back flow between chambers resulting in the noise. It was just a little smaller than a hole they would instantly operate on. She had no symptoms of struggling with anything so that was a blessing. We prayed like crazy and at a year later follow up they said it had closed completely! We were more than blessed to hear that.

Looking at her all you can see is a perfect little girl (and she is!) But, it's not a perfect world we live in. These two challenges are certainly not the last she will face. So, it's time to face reality. Life is not a fairy tale and neither is weight loss and health. There is no simple fix, if it looks too good to be true it is, and it's amazingly messy. Hopefully through our tiny families small struggles you can see fitness in a healthier though less clean and perfect kind of way. I hope this book will do the same for you while giving you tools to fight a good fight.

FIND US

www.talltrainer.com
Facebook: fb.me/talltrainer
Twitter: @talltrainer
Youtube: www.youtube.com/user/talltrainer
Email: 31lessons@talltrainer.com
Phone: 1(800)380-7047

Thank you for reading...

...God Bless!